SO-EIE-220

Praise for

The Glucose Revolution and The Glucose Revolution Pocket Guides

■

"The concept of the glycemic index has been distorted and bastardized by popular writers and diet gurus. Here, at last, is a book that explains what we know about the glycemic index and its importance in designing a diet for optimum health. Carbohydrates are not all bad. Read the good news about pasta and even—believe it or not—sugar!"
  —ANDREW WEIL, M.D., University of Arizona College of Medicine, author of *Spontaneous Healing* and *8 Weeks to Optimum Health*

■

"Forget *Sugar Busters*. Forget *The Zone*. If you want the real scoop on how carbohydrates and sugar affect your body, read this book by the world's leading researchers on the subject. It's the authoritative, last word on choosing foods to control your blood sugar."
  —JEAN CARPER, best-selling author of *Miracle Cures, Stop Aging Now!* and *Food: Your Miracle Medicine*

■

"Here is at last a book explaining the importance of taking into consideration the glycemic index of foods for overall health, athletic performance, and in reducing the risk of heart disease and diabetes. The book clearly explains that there are different kinds of carbohydrates

that work in different ways and why a universal recommendation to 'increase the carbohydrate content of your diet' is plainly simple and scientifically inaccurate. Everyone should put the glycemic index approach into practice."
—ARTEMIS P. SIMOPOULOS, M.D., senior author of *The Omega Diet* and *The Healing Diet* and President, The Center for Genetics, Nutrition and Health, Washington, D.C.

■

"*The Glucose Revolution* is nutrition science for the 21st century. Clearly written, it gives the scientific rationale for why all carbohydrates are not created equal. It is a practical guide for both professionals and patients. The food suggestions and recipes are exciting and tasty."
—RICHARD N. PODELL, M.D., M.P.H., Clinical Professor, Department of Family Medicine, UMDNJ–Robert Wood Johnson Medical School, and co-author of *The G-Index Diet: The Missing Link That Makes Permanent Weight Loss Possible*

■

"Although the jury is still out on the utility of the glycemic index, many of the curious will benefit from a careful reading of this book, and some will find that the glycemic index is particularly helpful for them. Everyone can enjoy the recipes, some of which are to die for!"
—JOHANNA DWYER, D. Sc.,R.D., editor, *Nutrition Today*

The Glucose Revolution Pocket Guide to
YOUR HEART

OTHER *GLUCOSE REVOLUTION* TITLES

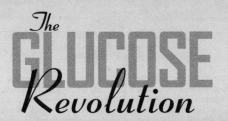

The GLUCOSE Revolution

POCKET GUIDE TO YOUR HEART

KAYE FOSTER-POWELL, M. NUTR. & DIET.

JENNIE BRAND-MILLER, PH.D.

ANTHONY LEEDS, M.D.

THOMAS M.S. WOLEVER, M.D., PH.D.

ADAPTED BY

JOHANNA BURANI, M.S., R.D., C.D.E.,

AND LINDA RAO, M.ED.

■

MARLOWE & COMPANY
NEW YORK

Published by
Marlowe & Company
841 Broadway, 4th Floor
New York, NY 10003

All rights reserved. No part of this book may be reproduced in whole or in part without written permission from the publishers, except by reviewers who may quote brief excerpts in connection with a review in a newspaper, magazine, or electronic publication; nor may any part of this book be reproduced, stored in a retrieval system, or transmitted in any form or by any means electronic, mechanical, photocopying, recording, or other, without written permission from the publisher.

The information in this book is intended to help readers make informed decisions about their health and the health of their loved ones. It is not intended to be a substitute for treatment by or the advice and care of a professional health care provider. While the authors and publisher have endeavored to ensure that the information is accurate and up to date, they are not responsible for adverse effects or consequences sustained by any person using this book.

Copyright © text 1998, 2000 Kaye Foster-Powell, Jennie Brand-Miller, Anthony Leeds, Thomas M. S. Wolever.

First published in Australia in 1999 in somewhat different form under the title *Pocket Guide to the G.I. Factor and Your Heart* by Hodder Headline Australia Pty Limited.

This edition is published by arrangement with Hodder Headline Australia Pty Limited.

Library of Congress Cataloging-in-Publication Data

Brand Miller, Janette, 1952-
    The glucose revolution pocket guide to your heart / Kaye Foster-Powell, Jennie Brand-Miller, Anthony Leeds, and Thomas M.S. Wolever.
        p   cm.
    ISBN 1-56924-640-8
    1. Heart—Diseases—Diet therapy.   2. Glycemic index.
3. Heart—Diseases—Prevention.   I. Title: Glucose revolution.
II. Fosster-Powell, Kaye.   III. Wolever, Thomas M.S. IV.
Title.

RC684.D5 B73 2000
616.1'20654—dc21

                                                                00-021901

9 8 7 6 5 4 3 2 1

Designed by Pauline Neuwirth, Neuwirth & Associates, Inc.
Distributed by Publishers Group West
Manufactured in the United States of America

CONTENTS

PREFACE

*T*he *Glucose Revolution* is the definitive, all-in-one guide to the glycemic index. Now we have written this pocket guide to show you how the glycemic index (G.I.) can help you control heart disease. As we explain in *The Glucose Revolution*, the glycemic index:

- is a proven guide to the true physiological effects foods—especially carbohydrates—have on blood sugar levels;
- provides an easy and effective way to eat a healthy diet and control fluctuations in blood sugar.

This book offers more in-depth information about using the glycemic index to prevent and control heart disease than we had room to include in *The Glucose Revolution*. Much new information appears in this book that is not in *The Glucose Revolution*, including a week's worth of low G.I. meal plans, as well as a success story about a man with heart disease who made the switch to low G.I. foods—and in the process achieved better control of his condition.

This book has been written to be read alongside *The Glucose Revolution*, so in the event you haven't already consulted that book, please be sure to do so, for a more comprehensive discussion of the glycemic index and all its uses.

Chapter 1

INTRODUCTION

A CLUSTER OF SYMPTOMS
THE GLYCEMIC INDEX AND HEART DISEASE

*H*eart disease is the single biggest killer of Americans. So big, in fact, that every 29 seconds an American will suffer either a heart attack or go into cardiac arrest. So what causes this deadly disease? It's often caused by atherosclerosis or "hardening of the arteries." Generally, people develop atherosclerosis gradually, and live much of their lives blissfully unaware of it. If the disease develops fairly slowly it may not cause any problems—even into great old age. But if its development is accelerated by one or more of many processes, the condition may cause trouble much earlier in life.

A CLUSTER OF SYMPTOMS

Heart disease seldom occurs as an isolated condition. For many years the medical profession has been aware that four major illnesses—heart disease, hypertension, obesity and diabetes—often occur together. This cluster of health problems occurs so frequently it has become known in the medical profession as Syndrome X. From a dietary perspective, experts have placed a lot of emphasis on the diet's fat content and how it influences these conditions, since high blood fat levels are a recognized characteristic of Syndrome X (see also page 34). While the type and amount of fat you eat is undoubtedly important to consider (as you'll read about later), newer research suggests that the type of *carbohydrate* plays a significant role, too.

The type of carbohydrate we eat determines the body's blood glucose response as well as the levels of insulin in our blood for many hours after we eat. We want to avoid the high insulin levels that occur when we eat foods with a high glycemic index. In the long term, higher insulin levels promote high blood fats, high blood pressure and increase heart attack risk.

Because of this, the diet's glycemic index is significant in the long-term prevention of heart disease and may be equally important to people who already have heart disease.

■

EATING A LOWER FAT DIET
WILL RESULT IN A HIGHER CARBOHYDRATE INTAKE.
WHAT MOST INFORMATION ON DIET AND HEART DISEASE
IGNORES IS THE IMPORTANCE OF THE
RIGHT TYPE OF CARBOHYDRATE.

■

THE GLYCEMIC INDEX AND HEART DISEASE

Most everyone these days is aware of the recommendations to cut back on fat to minimize our risk of heart disease. Very few people realize, however, that the type of carbohydrate we eat also influences our chances of developing not only heart disease, but also diabetes and obesity.

Did you know that:

- our intake of bread, potatoes, rice and pasta can influence our risk of heart disease?
- a diet rich in quickly digested carbohydrates may increase our risk of a heart attack?
- eating more fruit, whole grains, dried peas and beans and low fat dairy foods can reduce our risk of heart disease?

These are new findings from studies conducted during the 1990s that have important implications for the type of carbohydrate we eat.

Research on the *glycemic index* (G.I.) of foods shows that the type of carbohydrate we eat may have as much influence on our risk of heart disease as the type of fat we eat. Recent studies show that diets rich in slowly digested carbohydrates (with a low glycemic index):

- reduce blood cholesterol levels
- reduce "bad" LDL cholesterol
- increase "good" HDL cholesterol
- increase the body's sensitivity to insulin, and
- can help reduce body weight

■

DID YOU KNOW THAT A DIET RICH IN QUICKLY DIGESTED CARBOHYDRATES MAY INCREASE YOUR RISK OF A HEART ATTACK?

■

Chapter 2

TEST YOUR HEART KNOWLEDGE

TRUE/FALSE QUIZ

*B*efore we get into the subject of heart disease and the glycemic index in greater detail, take this quick quiz to test your knowledge. Answer true or false to the following questions.

True False

1. ___ ___ All vegetable oils are low in saturated fat.
2. ___ ___ Butter contains more fat than margarine.
3. ___ ___ Americans eat the recommended amount of fat.
4. ___ ___ You should avoid eggs on a low fat, cholesterol-lowering diet.

5. ___ ___ Moderate consumption of alcohol increases your risk of heart attack.
6. ___ ___ Olive oil is the lowest fat oil.
7. ___ ___ A cup of milk contains less fat than 2 squares of chocolate.
8. ___ ___ Nuts will raise cholesterol levels.
9. ___ ___ Potatoes and pasta are fattening foods.
10. ___ ___ Cod liver oil will lower cholesterol levels.

The answers to all the preceding questions are false. Here's why:

1. Contrary to popular belief, not all vegetable oils are low in saturated fat. Two primary exceptions are coconut oil and palm or palm kernel oil. Both these oils (which may appear on a food label simply as vegetable oil) are highly saturated. Palm oil is used widely in commercial cakes, biscuits, pastries and fried foods.
2. Butter and margarine contain similar levels of fat (around 85–90 percent). There is a difference in the types of fats that predominate, however; butter is about 60 percent saturated fat and unsaturated margarine is usually less than 30 percent saturated fat.
3. Americans get about 34 percent of their calories from fat. (The American Heart Association recommends no more than 30 percent of calories from fat for healthy people, and even less for people who have heart disease.) Unfortunately, we're gaining weight, too; most likely because we eat too many calorie-laden low fat and fat free snack foods.
4. Eggs are a source of cholesterol but dietary cholesterol tends to raise blood cholesterol levels

only when the rest of the diet is high in fat. One egg contains only about 5 grams of fat, of which only 2 grams is saturated.

5. Moderate amounts of alcohol (about two standard drinks per day) appear to reduce the risk of heart attack. Amounts in excess are harmful to health.

6. There is no such thing as low fat oil. Oil is 100 percent fat in a liquid form. Olive oil is a suitable choice of oils, since it contains only 15 percent saturated fats. Mediterranean populations, whose major source of fat is olive oil, have low levels of heart disease.

7. One cup (8 ounces) of whole milk contains 8 grams of fat. Compare this to about 4 grams contained in two small squares of chocolate!

8. Nuts have been found to be protective against heart disease. While most nuts are high in fat, much of the fat they contain is of the "good" unsaturated type.

9. This is a myth that has been around for years. Potato and pasta are high carbohydrate foods, which means they're both good sources of energy for the body. They are rarely stored as body fat.

10. Cod liver oil has not been found to lower cholesterol levels. It is extremely rich in vitamins A and D and should not be taken in large doses because of the danger of vitamin A toxicity.

Chapter 3

THE GLYCEMIC INDEX: SOME BACKGROUND

HOW THE MILLS CHANGED EVERYTHING

HOW THE GLYCEMIC INDEX CAME TO BE

EARLY CRITICISM

WHAT IS THE GLYCEMIC INDEX?

THE GLYCEMIC INDEX MADE SIMPLE

MEASURING THE GLYCEMIC INDEX

For the past 10,000 years, our ancestors survived on a high carbohydrate and low fat diet. They ate their carbohydrates in the form of beans, vegetables and whole cereal grains, and got their sugars from fibrous fruits and berries. Food preparation was a simple process: They ground food between stones and cooked it over the heat of an open fire. The result? All of their food was digested and absorbed slowly, which raised their blood sugar levels more slowly and over a longer period of time.

This diet was ideal for their bodies because it provided slow release energy that helped to delay hunger pangs and provided fuel for working muscles long after the meal was eaten. The slow rise in blood sugar was also kind to the pancreas, the organ that produces insulin.

HOW THE MILLS CHANGED EVERYTHING

As time passed, flours were ground more and more finely and bran was separated completely from the white flour. With the advent of high speed roller mills in the nineteenth century, it was possible to produce white flour so fine that it resembled talcum powder in appearance and texture. These fine white flours have always been highly prized because they make soft bread and light, airy sponge cakes. As incomes grew, people pushed their peas and beans aside and started eating more meat. As a consequence, the composition of the average diet changed, in that we began to eat more fat and because the type of carbohydrate in our diet changed, it became more quickly digested and absorbed. Something we didn't expect happened, too: The blood sugar rise after a meal was higher and more prolonged, stimulating the pancreas to produce more insulin.

THE PANCREAS PRODUCES INSULIN

The pancreas is a vital organ near the stomach, and its main job is to produce the hormone insulin. Carbohydrate stimulates the secretion of insulin more than any other component of food. The slow absorption of the carbohydrate in our food means that the pancreas doesn't have to work so hard and needs to produce less insulin. If the pancreas is overstimulated over a long period of time, it may become "exhausted" and type 2 diabetes can develop in genetically susceptible people. Even without diabetes, high insulin levels are undesirable because they increase the risk of heart disease.

Unfortunately, over time, we have begun to eat more "refined" foods and fewer "whole" foods. This new way of eating has brought with it higher blood sugar levels after a meal and higher insulin responses, as well. Though our bodies do need insulin for carbohydrate metabolism, high levels of the hormone have a profound effect on the development of many diseases. In fact, medical experts now believe that high insulin levels are one of the key factors responsible for heart disease and hypertension. Insulin influences the way we metabolize foods, determining whether we burn fat or carbohydrate to meet our energy needs and ultimately determining whether we store fat in our bodies.

HOW THE GLYCEMIC INDEX CAME TO BE

The glycemic index concept was first developed in 1981 by a team of scientists led by Dr. David Jenkins, a professor of nutrition at the University of Toronto, Canada, to help determine which foods were best for people with diabetes. At that time, the diet for people with diabetes was based on a system of carbohydrate exchanges or portions, which was complicated and not very logical. The carbohydrate exchange system assumed that all starchy foods produce the same effect on blood sugar levels even though some earlier studies had already proven this was not correct. Jenkins was one of the first researchers to question this assumption and to investigate how real foods behave in the bodies of real people.

Jenkins's approach attracted a great deal of attention because it was so logical and systematic. He and his colleagues had tested a large number of common foods, and some of their results were surprising. Ice cream, for example, despite its sugar content, had much less effect on blood sugar than some ordinary breads. Over the next 15 years medical researchers and scientists around the world, including the authors of this book, tested the effect of many foods on blood sugar levels and developed a new concept of classifying carbohydrates based on their glycemic index.

WHAT IS THE GLYCEMIC INDEX?

The glycemic index of foods is simply a ranking of foods based on their immediate effect on blood sugar levels. To make a fair comparison, all foods are compared with a reference food such as pure glucose and are tested in equivalent carbohydrate amounts.

Originally, research into the glycemic index of foods was inspired by the desire to identify the best foods for people with diabetes. But scientists are now discovering that G.I. values have implications for everyone.

Today we know the glycemic index of hundreds of different food items—both generic and name-brand—that have been tested following a standardized testing method. The tables in Chapter 19 on pages 91 to 103 give the glycemic index of a range of common foods, including many tested at the University of Toronto and the University of Sydney.

■ ■ ■

THE GLYCEMIC INDEX MADE SIMPLE

Carbohydrate foods that break down quickly during digestion have the highest G.I. values. The blood glucose, or sugar, response is fast and high. In other words the glucose in the bloodstream increases rapidly. Conversely, carbohydrates that break down slowly, releasing glucose gradually into the bloodstream, have low G.I. values. An analogy might be the popular fable of the tortoise and the hare. The hare, just like high G.I. foods, speeds away full steam ahead but loses the race to the tortoise with his slow and steady pace. Similarly, slow and steady low G.I. foods produce a smooth blood sugar curve without wild fluctuations.

For most people most of the time, the foods with a low glycemic index have advantages over those with high G.I. values. Figure 1 shows the effect of slow and fast carbohydrate on blood sugar levels (Figure 1).

The substance that produces the greatest rise in blood sugar levels is pure glucose itself. All other foods have less effect when fed in equal amounts of carbohydrate. The glycemic index of pure glucose is set at 100, and every other food is ranked on a scale from 0 to 100 according to its actual effect on blood sugar levels.

The glycemic index of a food cannot be predicted from its composition or the glycemic index of related foods. To test the glycemic index, you need real people and real foods. (We describe how the glycemic index of a food is measured below.) There is no easy, inexpensive substitute test. Scientists always follow standardized methods so that results from one group of people can be directly compared with those of another group.

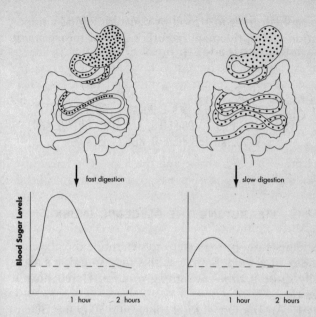

Figure1. Slow and fast carbohydrate digestion and the consequent levels of sugar in the blood.

In total, 8 to 10 people need to be tested and the glycemic index of the food is the average value of the group. We know this average figure is reproducible and that a different group of volunteers will produce a similar result. Results obtained in a group of people with diabetes are comparable to those without diabetes.

The most important point to note is that all foods are tested in equivalent carbohydrate amounts. For example, 100 grams of bread (about 3½ slices of sandwich bread) is tested because this contains 50 grams of carbohydrate. Likewise, 60 grams of jelly beans (containing 50 grams of carbohydrate) is compared with the reference food. We know how much

carbohydrate is in a food by consulting food composition tables, the manufacturer's data or measuring it
ourselves in the laboratory.

■

THE GLYCEMIC INDEX IS A CLINICALLY PROVEN TOOL IN ITS APPLICATIONS TO DIABETES, APPETITE CONTROL AND REDUCING THE RISK OF HEART DISEASE.

■

MEASURING THE GLYCEMIC INDEX

Scientists use just six steps to determine the glycemic
index of a food. Simple as this may sound, it's actually quite a time-consuming process. Here's how it
works.

1. An amount of food containing 50 grams of carbohydrate is given to a volunteer to eat. For example,
to test boiled spaghetti, the volunteer would be given
200 grams of spaghetti, which supplies 50 grams of
carbohydrate (we work this out from food composition tables or by measuring the available carbohydrate)—50 grams of carbohydrate is equivalent to 3
tablespoons of pure glucose powder.

2. Over the next two hours (or three hours if the
volunteer has diabetes), we take a sample of their
blood every 15 minutes during the first hour and
thereafter every 30 minutes. The blood sugar level of
these blood samples is measured in the laboratory
and recorded.

3. The blood sugar level is plotted on a graph and
the area under the curve is calculated using a com-
puter program (Figure 2).

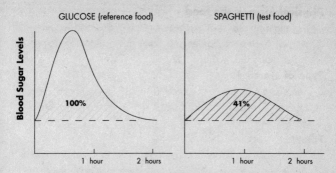

Figure 2. The effect of pure glucose (50 g) and spaghetti (50 g carbohydrate portion) on blood sugar levels.

4. The volunteer's response to spaghetti (or whatever food is being tested) is compared with his or her blood sugar response to 50 grams of pure glucose (the reference food).

5. The reference food is tested on two or three separate occasions and an average value is calculated. This is done to reduce the effect of day-to-day variation in blood sugar responses.

6. The average glycemic index found in 8 to 10 people is the glycemic index of that food.

---

5 KEY FACTORS THAT INFLUENCE THE GLYCEMIC INDEX

Cooking methods

Cooking and processing increases the glycemic index of a food because it increases the amount of gelatinized starch in the food. Corn flakes is one example.

Physical form of the food

An intact fibrous coat, such as that on grains and legumes, acts as a physical barrier and slows down digestion, lowering a food's G.I. value.

Type of starch

There are two types of starch in foods, amylose and amylopectin. The more amylose starch a food contains, the lower the glycemic index.

Fiber

Viscous, soluble fibers, such as those found in rolled oats and apples, slow down digestion and lower a food's glycemic index.

Sugar

The presence of sugar, as well as the type of sugar, will influence a food's glycemic index. Fruits with a low glycemic index, such as apples and oranges, are high in fructose.

Chapter 4

THE PROCESS OF
ATHEROSCLEROSIS

HOW THROMBOSIS OCCURS

WHY DO PEOPLE GET HEART DISEASE?

*A*therosclerosis results in reduced blood flow through the blood vessels, which can mean that the heart muscle gets insufficient oxygen to provide the power for pumping blood. That, in turn, can cause angina pectoris (pain in the central chest). Elsewhere in the body, atherosclerosis has a similar blood-flow-reducing effect: In the legs, atherosclerosis can cause muscle pains when you exercise (called intermittent claudication); and in the brain it can cause a variety of problems, including strokes.

An even more serious consequence of atherosclerosis occurs when a blood clot forms over the surface of a patch of atherosclerosis on an artery. This

process, called *thrombosis*, can completely block an
artery, resulting in small heart attacks or even sudden
death.

HOW THROMBOSIS OCCURS

The process of thrombosis can occur elsewhere in the
arteries, as well; the consequences of which are determined by the extent of the thrombosis. Whether you
develop thrombosis depends in large part on the tendency of the blood to clot versus the blood's natural
ability to break down clots. (These two counteracting
tendencies are influenced by a number of factors,
including some dietary factors, most notably the
effect of fatty fish or fish oils in the diet. We'll discuss
this in more detail in "10 Tips to a Heart-Healthy,
Low G.I. Diet" on page 41.)

Those people who suffer from coronary (heart)
artery atherosclerosis may slowly develop reduced
heart function. For a while the heart may be able to
compensate for the problem, so there may be no
symptoms, but eventually it will begin to fail. You
may experience shortness of breath when you first
start to exercise, and sometimes your ankles may
swell. Atherosclerosis can also lead to an abnormal
heart beat (palpitations). Remember that your heart
isn't the only part of your body that may be affected:
You may also notice poor leg circulation, which can
make your legs and feet feel cold, and exercise may
be painful. If your brain doesn't get enough blood
due to the poor circulation, you may also be susceptible to a "mini" or even a major stroke.

Modern medicine has many effective drug treatments for heart failure, so this consequence of ather

osclerosis doesn't have quite the same serious implications as it did in the past.

WHY DO PEOPLE GET HEART DISEASE?

For most people atherosclerotic heart disease develops gradually over a number of years. The process
begins early in life and is influenced by many factors
to which a person is exposed. Over the past few
decades doctors and scientists have identified in fine
detail the processes that cause heart disease, so they
are well aware of most of the factors that contribute
to the disease.

Theoretically, atherosclerotic heart disease might
be largely prevented if researchers were able to assess
everyone's risks during childhood and could encour-
age them to do all the "right" things throughout the
rest of their lives. In practice, though, there's been
limited development of the ways to screen people
early in life for their heart disease risk, and the
resources needed to achieve large scale prevention are
just not available.

A great deal is known, however, about the risk factors for heart disease and those who heed the information and take the necessary action can reduce their
risk. We discuss the risk factors for heart disease on
pages 23 to 28.

Chapter 5

HOW CAN THE GLYCEMIC INDEX HELP?

PRIMARY AND SECONDARY PREVENTION

HEALTH CHECKS AND LIFESTYLE ADVICE

*W*e know from early research that the glycemic index may reduce the risk of heart disease by helping to reduce body weight and improving blood glucose control. What later research has shown is that the glycemic index of the diet has further reaching effects on our risk of heart disease. Low G.I. diets also reduce total blood cholesterol and low density (LDL) cholesterol in some people (lower levels of total cholesterol and LDL cholesterol are associated with a lower risk of heart disease).

Interestingly, in addition to these effects, low G.I. diets may influence the "good" cholesterol in blood—that is the high-density (HDL) cholesterol.

HDL cholesterol is a marker of the body moving cholesterol away from arteries, so the higher the number, the better. Large scale surveys have shown that high HDL cholesterol is also associated with a lower risk of heart disease.

A study of the diets of over a thousand people in Britain showed that those who followed a low G.I. diet had significantly higher HDL cholesterol levels than those who did not. In addition, preliminary reports here in the United States showed that when diet and risk of heart disease were followed for several years in many thousands of women, the risk of heart disease was found to be lower in those who had eaten a low G.I. diet. This effect may be because low G.I. diets affect the body's sensitivity to insulin (see page 34), which in turn increases levels of HDL cholesterol.

The glycemic index may also reduce the risk of heart disease by helping to reduce body weight and improving blood glucose control.

PRIMARY AND SECONDARY PREVENTION

When doctors detect heart disease, they have two treatment options available, depending on the state of the disease. First, they treat the effects of the disease (such as with medical treatment with drugs and surgical treatment to bypass blocked arteries) and second, they address the risk factors involved to help slow down further progression of the disease.

Treatment of risk factors after the disease has already developed is called "secondary prevention." In people who have not yet developed the disease, treatment of risk factors is called "primary prevention."

Obviously it would be better to give primary preventive treatment in all cases but luckily, the glycemic index has applications in both cases.

HEALTH CHECKS AND LIFESTYLE ADVICE

More and more people now get regular checks of their blood pressure and blood fats, as well as tests to check for diabetes. All health professionals give patients lifestyle advice to help them stop smoking, exercise more and eat a good diet. When doctors discover specific risk factors, they give diet and lifestyle advice, but sometimes patients don't follow this advice for very long.

It's especially difficult for patients to follow advice if they aren't likely to feel any ill effects of not following that advice for 10 or more years, and if the changes they need to make are hard to stick to. The person must want to make certain changes and must get support from friends and relatives to keep at it. Also, it's preferable if the person sees the changes in a positive light, thinking to themselves, "I want to do this," instead of "My doctor told me to do this." Any new dimension in heart disease prevention must be seen as a great positive change rather than as a negative one.

Chapter 6

HEART DISEASE RISK FACTORS

SMOKING

HIGH BLOOD PRESSURE

DIABETES

HIGH CHOLESTEROL

HIGH CHOLESTEROL FOODS

LACK OF EXERCISE

*Y*our chance of developing heart disease is increased if you smoke tobacco, have high blood pressure, diabetes or high blood cholesterol (which may be because you eat too much fat), or if you're overweight or obese or if you don't get enough physical exercise.

SMOKING

Smoking of tobacco is now clearly established as a cause of atherosclerosis; few authorities dispute the evidence. There are, however, some interesting dietary aspects that go along with this risk factor:

Did you know that smokers:

- tend to eat fewer servings of fruits and vegetables compared to non-smokers (and consequently eat fewer protective antioxidants)?
- tend to eat more fat and more salt than non-smokers?

It could be that smokers eat fewer fruits and veggies and more fat because their tastebuds have been blunted by the smoking and they're seeking stronger flavors. Because these dietary differences may put the smoker at greater risk of heart disease there is only one piece of advice for anyone who smokes:

■

PLEASE STOP SMOKING!

■

HIGH BLOOD PRESSURE

High blood pressure killed more than 40,000 Americans in 1996. Recent estimates suggest that 25 percent of U.S. adults have high blood pressure, but because hypertension has no symptoms, more than one-third of these people don't even know they have it! High blood pressure (hypertension) is very damaging because it makes your heart work harder and damages your arteries. Remember, an artery is not a rigid pipe: It's a muscular tube, which, when healthy, can change its size to control blood flow.

High blood pressure causes changes in the artery walls that makes atherosclerosis more likely to develop.

Blood clots can then form and the weakened blood vessels can easily rupture and bleed.

Treatments for blood pressure have become more effective over the last 30 years, but it's only now becoming clear which types of treatment for blood pressure are also effective at reducing heart disease risk.

■

OPTIMAL BLOOD PRESSURE (AS IT RELATES TO HEART DISEASE) IS LESS THAN 120/80.

■

DIABETES

Diabetes is, in itself, a further risk factor for heart disease. Diabetes is caused by a lack of insulin— either the body doesn't produce enough, or the body demands more than normal (because it has become insensitive to insulin). In diabetes some of the chemical (metabolic) processes that take place also tend to accelerate atherosclerosis. Diabetes may also cause an increase in blood fats, which is an independent risk factor for heart disease.

The increased risk of heart disease is a major reason why doctors and other health professionals put so much effort into helping diabetic patients achieve blood sugar control. It's also why all people with diabetes should be checked for the other risk factors of heart disease.

For more information about how the glycemic index can be used to manage diabetes, see *The Glucose Revolution Pocket Guide to Diabetes*.

HIGH CHOLESTEROL

High blood cholesterol also increases your risk of heart disease. Your blood cholesterol is determined by genetic (inherited) factors—which you can't change—and lifestyle factors—which you *can* change. There are also some relatively rare genetic conditions that can cause particularly high blood cholesterol levels.

People who have inherited these conditions need a thorough workup by a specialist, followed by life-long drug treatment. In most people high blood cholesterol is partly determined by their genes, which have "set" the cholesterol levels slightly high to begin with, plus lifestyle factors, which push the numbers up even more. Body weight also affects blood cholesterol—in some people being overweight has a significant effect on cholesterol levels—so reaching (and maintaining) a reasonable weight can be helpful. The most important dietary factor is fat, and in particular, saturated fat. Some sources of saturated fat include whole milk, cream, cheese, ice cream, butter, red meats, coconut and palm oils and chocolate.

To lower blood cholesterol levels, experts recommend low fat (low saturated fat), high carbohydrate, high fiber diets. The blood also contains triglycerides, another type of fat that may be linked with increased risk of heart disease in some people. Levels of both cholesterol and triglycerides need to be checked as part of your heart disease risk assessment.

■

YOUR BLOOD CHOLESTEROL IS DETERMINED BY GENETIC
(INHERITED) FACTORS—WHICH YOU CANNOT
CHANGE—AND LIFESTYLE FACTORS—WHICH YOU
CAN CHANGE.

■

HIGH CHOLESTEROL FOODS

Many people who aim to lower their risk of heart disease focus on avoiding high-cholesterol foods. Unfortunately, this approach puts the emphasis in the wrong place. Cholesterol itself is concentrated in very few foods (see below) and is not the main cause of our high blood cholesterol levels. In fact, the amount of cholesterol we obtain from food is generally much less than the amount of cholesterol our body makes on its own. Our body can make all the cholesterol we need, but in certain circumstances, we make more than we need, which causes our blood cholesterol levels to build up and become a problem.

Those foods that do contain a good deal of cholesterol include:

- Liver and kidney
- Egg yolk
- Caviar

A diet high in saturated fat is one of the contributors to high blood cholesterol. Reducing saturated fat intake can usually improve cholesterol levels. See "High cholesterol" on page 26 for some dietary sources of saturated fat.

LACK OF EXERCISE

Lack of exercise also increases the risk of heart disease. Our cardiovascular fitness improves when we get regular, strenuous exercise (the blood supply to the heart may improve at the same time). Specifically, cardiovascular fitness is improved by *aerobic* exercise, which is activity that makes your heart beat faster so your pulse increases and you breathe more deeply.

Experts believe that we need to accumulate at least 30 minutes each day of this level of exertion to maintain cardiovascular fitness. Exercise is also important in maintaining body weight and has effects on metabolism and some factors related to blood clotting. Clearly, getting regular exercise is important. So don't just think about it, just do it! (For more information about the importance of exercise, see Chapter 9, "Exercise: We Can't Live Without It" on page 37.)

Chapter 7

OBESITY AND HEART DISEASE

WHAT'S YOUR SHAPE?

WHY DIETS DON'T WORK

QUANTITY ISN'T THE ISSUE—
THE GLYCEMIC INDEX IS

THERE'S NO NEED TO FEEL HUNGRY
WHEN YOU'RE LOSING WEIGHT

*O*besity is one of the biggest risk factors for heart disease. And though it seems as if everyone is on a diet these days, the number of overweight and obese people in our society is actually *climbing*! In fact, during the 1990s alone, the number of adult Americans has grown by what some experts are calling epidemic proportions: almost 50 percent! (The number of obese people in the state of Georgia, for example, has grown more than 100 percent over the past decade.)

The problem is so pervasive that some studies find 55 percent of American adults weighing more than they should, and 33 percent of these people are actually obese. (Twenty-five percent of all U.S. children are overweight, too.) A half million people die every year from excess weight.

If this trend continues, experts say that within just a few generations, *every adult American* will be overweight! Clearly, to bring heart disease under control, we need to get our weight under control.

■

SOME STUDIES SHOW THAT 55 PERCENT OF AMERICAN ADULTS WEIGH MORE THAN THEY SHOULD.

■

NO LAUGHING MATTER

One study, conducted at St. Luke's/Roosevelt Medical Center in New York City, found that 325,000 deaths in the U.S. each year can be attributed to obesity. That makes obesity the *second leading cause of preventable death*—surpassed only by smoking.

America's weight problem isn't surprising, you may think, given the abundance of foods available to us. We eat away from home more often than we used to and consume greater amounts of fast and snack foods than ever before. As a nation, we were doing better for a while, when reported intakes of fat and calories were going down, but new research shows that the trend for fat consumption is now drifting back up.

■　■　■

WHAT'S YOUR SHAPE?

Fat around the middle part of our body (abdominal fat) increases our risk of heart disease, high blood pressure and diabetes. In contrast, fat on the lower part of the body, such as on our hips and thighs doesn't carry the same health risk. Your body shape can be described according to your distribution of body fat as either an "apple" or a "pear" shape (Figure 3).

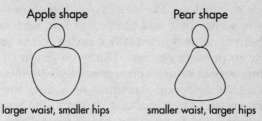

Apple shape   Pear shape

larger waist, smaller hips   smaller waist, larger hips

Figure 3. There is significant health benefit in reducing your waist measurement, particularly if you can have an 'apple' shape.

You can easily tell if you are an apple or a pear by taking a tape measure around your waist and then your hips and seeing which is smaller. (Ideally the waist is smaller than the hips.)

Specifically, the ratio (your waist measurement divided by your hip measurement) between the two should be:

- less than 0.9 for men, and
- less than 0.8 for women

WHY DIETS DON'T WORK

If you are overweight (or consider yourself to be) chances are that you have looked at countless books, brochures and magazines offering a solution to losing weight. New diets or miracle weight-loss solutions seem to appear weekly. They are clearly good for selling magazines, but for the majority of people who are overweight "diets" just don't work (if they did, there wouldn't be so many!).

At best, a "diet" will reduce your calorie intake. At worst, it will change your body composition for the fatter. The reason? Many diets teach you to reduce your carbohydrate intake to bring about quick weight loss. The weight you lose, however, is mostly water (that was trapped or held with stored carbohydrate) and eventually muscle (as it is broken down to produce glucose). Once you return to your former way of eating, you regain a little bit more fat. With each desperate repetition of a diet, you lose more muscle. Over a course of years, the resultant change in body composition to less muscle and more fat makes it increasingly difficult to lose weight.

■

FOR THE MAJORITY OF PEOPLE WHO ARE OVERWEIGHT, MAGAZINE "MIRACLE DIETS" DON'T WORK. IF THEY DID, THERE WOULDN'T BE SO MANY OF THEM.

■

QUANTITY ISN'T THE ISSUE —THE GLYCEMIC INDEX IS

Low G.I. foods have two very special advantages for people who want to lose weight: They fill you up and keep you satisfied for longer, and they help you burn more of your body fat and less of your body muscle.

If you're trying to lose weight, low G.I. foods will enable you to increase your food intake without increasing your waistline, control your appetite and choose the right carbohydrates for your lifestyle and your well-being.

THERE'S NO NEED TO FEEL HUNGRY WHEN YOU'RE LOSING WEIGHT

When you use the glycemic index as the basis for your food choices, you *DON'T* need to overly restrict your food intake, obsessively count calories or starve yourself. That way, you can lose weight (and reduce your risk of heart disease) *without* feeling hungry!

Chapter 8

THE GLYCEMIC INDEX
AND INSULIN
SENSITIVITY

WHAT THE RESEARCH SHOWS

LOW G.I. DIETS IMPROVE RISK FACTORS

*C*onditions such as high blood pressure, excess weight or obesity, diabetes, or high blood fats rarely occur in isolation. Many people have a cluster of these conditions, which we referred to earlier as Syndrome X. Syndrome X is characterized by high blood sugar levels, high blood fat levels (especially triglycerides), excess weight, high blood pressure, increased blood clotting and high blood insulin levels. We know that people with this condition become *insensitive* to insulin.

The tissues of the body change so that the body needs more insulin to achieve the same effect as usual, and the body responds by circulating more insulin in the blood. Tests on patients with heart disease show that a higher-than-expected number of these people have an insensitivity to insulin.

WHAT THE RESEARCH SHOWS

Can a low G.I. diet help? In a recent study, patients with serious coronary artery disease were given either low or high G.I. diets before surgery for coronary bypass grafts. They were given blood tests before their diets and just before surgery, and during their surgery, doctors removed small pieces of fat tissue for testing.

The tests on the fat showed that the low G.I. diets made the tissues of these "insulin-insensitive" patients more sensitive to the hormone—in fact, they were back in the same range as normal control patients after just a few weeks on the low G.I. diet!

If people with serious heart disease can improve, would the same happen with younger people? Researchers tried to answer this question when they divided young women in their thirties into two groups: those who did and those who did not have a family history of heart disease. (The women themselves had not yet developed the condition.) After a series of blood tests, the women followed either a low or high G.I. diet for four weeks, after which they had more blood tests. Then, during surgeries unrelated to heart disease, doctors removed pieces of fat and tested them for insulin sensitivity. The young women with a family history of heart disease were insensitive to insulin originally (those without the family history of heart disease were normal), but after four weeks on the low G.I. diet their insulin sensitivity was normal.

In both studies the diets were designed to try to ensure that all the other variables (total energy, total carbohydrates) were not different, so that the change in insulin sensitivity the researchers found was likely to have been due to the low G.I. diet rather than any other factor.

LOW G.I. DIETS IMPROVE RISK FACTORS

Work on these exciting findings continues, but what we know so far strongly suggests that low G.I. diets not only improve body weight and improve blood sugar in people with diabetes, but also the body's insulin sensitivity. It will take many years of further research to show that this simple dietary change to a low G.I. diet will definitely slow the progress of atherosclerotic heart disease, of course, but in the meantime it's clear that heart disease risk factors improve on a low G.I. diet. By the way, low G.I. diets are consistent with the other required dietary changes needed to help prevent heart disease.

■

THE MESSAGE FOR HEART DISEASE PREVENTION: EAT A LOW FAT (LOW SATURATED FAT), HIGH CARBOHYDRATE, HIGH FIBER, LOW G.I. DIET!

■

Chapter 9

EXERCISE: WE CAN'T LIVE WITHOUT IT

THE BENEFITS OF EXERCISE

HOW TO GET MOVING

8 WAYS TO MAKE EXERCISE WORK FOR YOU

A multitude of changes in living habits now mean that in both work and recreation we are more sedentary. Unfortunately, sedentary lifestyles lead to excess weight, which can, in turn, increase your risk of heart disease. Our physical activity levels are now so low that we have an imbalance in our energy equation so that we don't burn up enough calories to account for the amount we eat.

■

TO LOSE WEIGHT YOU NEED TO EAT FEWER CALORIES AND BURN MORE CALORIES——AND THAT MEANS GETTING REGULAR EXERCISE AND LEADING A MORE ACTIVE LIFESTYLE.

■

THE BENEFITS OF EXERCISE

Most people could tell you at least one health benefit of exercise (reduces blood pressure, lowers the risk of heart disease, improves circulation, increases stamina, flexibility and strength), but the most motivating aspect of exercise is feeling so good about yourself for doing it.

Exercise speeds up our metabolic rate. By increasing our caloric expenditure, exercise helps to balance our sometimes excessive caloric intake from food.

More movement makes our muscles better at using fat as a source of fuel. By improving the way insulin works, exercise increases the amount of fat we burn.

A low G.I. diet has the same effect. Low G.I. foods reduce the amount of insulin we need, which makes fat easier to burn and harder to store. Since it's body fat that you want to get rid of when you lose weight, exercise in combination with a low G.I. diet makes a lot of sense!

HOW TO GET MOVING

Getting more exercise doesn't necessarily mean daily aerobics classes and jogging around the block (although this is great if you want to do it). What it *does* mean is moving more in everyday living. It's the day-to-day things we do—shopping, ironing, chasing kids, walking from the train station—where we spend the bulk of our energy. Since so much of our lifestyle is designed now to reduce our physical exertion, it's become very important to catch bursts of physical activity wherever we can, to increase our energy output. It may mean using the stairs instead of the elevator, taking a 10 minute walk at lunch time, trotting on a treadmill while you watch the news or talk on the telephone, walking to the grocery store to get the Sunday paper, hiding the remote control, parking a half-mile from work or taking the dog for a walk each night. Whatever it means, do it. Even housework burns calories!

HOW EXERCISE KEEPS YOU MOVING

The effect of exercise doesn't stop when you do. People who exercise have higher metabolic rates, so their bodies continue to burn more calories every minute, even when they're asleep!

Besides increasing your incidental activity you will also benefit from some planned aerobic activity, which causes you to breathe more heavily and makes your heart beat faster. Walking, cycling, swimming and stair climbing are just a few examples. You'll need to accumulate a total of at least 30 minutes of this type of activity 5 to 6 days a week.

■

EXERCISE MAKES OUR MUSCLES BETTER AT USING FAT AS A SOURCE OF FUEL.

■

Remember that reduction in body weight takes time. Even after you've made changes in your exercise habits, your weight may not be any different on the scales. This is particularly true in women, whose bodies tend to adapt to increased caloric expenditure.

Whatever it takes for you to burn more calories, do it. Try to regard movement as an opportunity to improve your physical well being—not as an inconvenience.

8 WAYS TO MAKE EXERCISE WORK FOR YOU

Your exercise routine will bring you lots of benefits if you can:

1. See how it benefits you.
2. Enjoy what you do.
3. Feel that you can do it fairly well.
4. Fit it in with your daily life.
5. Keep it inexpensive.
6. Make it accessible.
7. Stay safe while doing it.
8. Make it socially acceptable to your peers.

Chapter 10

10 TIPS FOR A HEART-HEALTHY, LOW G.I. DIET

PICK MORE WHOLE GRAINS

CHOOSE BEANS, PEAS AND LENTILS

STRIVE FOR FIVE

EAT OILY FISH TWICE A WEEK

MINIMIZE SATURATED FATS

REDUCE SALT

MODERATE ALCOHOL

INCLUDE NUTS

CHOOSE LOW FAT DAIRY

HAVE A TREAT

1. FEAST ON MORE WHOLE GRAINS

Whole cereal grains represent what were the earliest forms of cereal for humans. Eaten boiled or roughly pounded to a flour, mixed with water and roasted, they were a form of slow-release carbohydrate with a low glycemic index, and they were also filling and sustaining. The advent of high speed roller mills during the Industrial Revolution led to the development of the fine, white flour that we use today. Because the outer seed coat has been removed, the starch in today's flour is readily digested and has a high glycemic index.

But we can still get the benefit of whole grains in our diet today with foods such as:

- Barley—such as pearled barley in soup
- Whole wheat or cracked wheat (bulgur)
- Oats and rolled oats for breakfast
- Whole grain breads (the ones with chewy grains and seeds)
- 100% stoneground whole wheat bread
- Whole grain pumpernickel
- Natural Ovens 100% Whole Grain**

If you're making your own bread, you can add your own G.I. lowering ingredients, such as linseed, flaxseed, rolled oats, cornmeal, oat bran, barley meal, cracked wheat and wheat berries.

**Natural Ovens ordering information appears in the "For More Information" section at the back of this book.

2. USE MORE DRIED BEANS, PEAS AND LENTILS

Dried peas, beans and lentils are collectively known as legumes. These are excellent foods that are:
- rich in low G.I. carbohydrate
- low in fat
- high in fiber
- low in cost

Because they are high in protein, legumes are an ideal substitute for meat. Introduce them to your family gradually by incorporating them in meals with meat such as in chili con carne, a filling for tacos or burritos, and in soups and salads. You can also try some of the delicious vegetarian dishes made with legumes.

It's easy to use legumes in soups and chili, but have you thought about:

- a mixed 3-bean salad
- a can of kidney beans in a spaghetti meat sauce
- hummus dip or spread
- ham and split pea soup

Legume products to look for:

- canned soups with lentils, chick peas and kidney beans (such as Healthy Choice or Health Valley)
- canned baked beans, kidney beans, butter beans, soy beans
- any variety of dried peas or beans (Goya is a major manufacturer of bean products)

THE SPECIAL BENEFIT OF SOY

Foods based on soy beans also have a beneficial role in our defense against heart disease. There are two components of soy beans with the potential to reduce coronary heart disease risk: soy protein and antioxidant substances called isoflavones.

Soy foods:

- improve our blood fats—lowering the bad (LDL cholesterol and triglyceride) and increasing the good (HDL cholesterol)
- reduce the accumulation of cholesterol in blood vessels by decreasing LDL oxidation

- decrease the tendency to form blood clots or thromboses
- have health promoting effects on blood vessels

Studies suggest that one to two servings of soy-protein-rich food each day may be sufficient to provide long-term health benefits. Just 1 cup of soy milk constitutes a serving and can be used as a nutritionally balanced replacement for dairy milk, as long as it's fortified with calcium. Try:

- soy milk on your breakfast cereal
- a soy milk and banana smoothie

3. EAT LOTS OF FRUITS AND VEGETABLES

Plant foods are rich sources of naturally occurring chemicals believed to be involved in disease prevention. Increased consumption of fruit and vegetables is associated with a lower incidence of diseases such as cancer, cardiovascular disease and other age-related diseases.

Health experts recommend that you strive to eat at least five servings a day of fruit and vegetables. These foods are an essential source of vitamin C but are also rich in antioxidants and fiber.

Get into a fruit and vegetable habit by:

- including fruits and veggies in all of your main meals
- taking an apple and a banana to work
- preparing one vegetarian meal each week
- making a habit of eating some fruit at home when you relax in the evening

- ordering a side salad with your meal
- preparing a fruit platter for the household to share after the meal
- buying a new vegetable to try each week
- considering fresh, canned, dried and juiced fruit as sources of fruit for your diet
- chopping fresh pineapple or melon into large chunks and keeping it on hand in the refrigerator
- preparing large amounts of vegetable soups and sauces and freeze in family or individual portions to use later

4. EAT OILY FISH AT LEAST TWICE A WEEK

Oily fish are the best source of long chain omega-3 fatty acids. These types of fats are scarcely found in other foods and offer valuable benefits in reducing blood clotting and inflammatory reactions. They can help in the prevention and treatment of heart disease, high blood pressure and rheumatoid arthritis. They are also beneficial in infant brain and eye development.

Fresh fish that are highest in omega-3 fats include:

- Swordfish
- Atlantic salmon
- Silver perch
- Mackerel

Canned fish can also provide substantial amounts of omega-3 fats. Good sources include:

- Mackerel

- Salmon
- Sardines

Smoked salmon is also an excellent source.

■

AIM TO EAT A TYPE OF OILY FISH AT LEAST TWICE A
WEEK AS A MAIN MEAL (JUST DON'T FRY FRESH FISH IN
SATURATED FAT).

■

5. REDUCE SATURATED FATS

Americans eat too much fat in general. Saturated fat,
in particular, is believed to be a major cause of high
cholesterol levels.

The main sources are:

- whole milk dairy foods, including cheese and
  cream
- frozen desserts such as ice cream
- meat, especially processed meats such as
  sausage, salami and hot dogs
- high-fat cold cuts including bologna and liverwurst
- fat spreads, especially butter, cream cheese and
  cheese spreads (the exception: natural peanut
  butter)
- takeout foods, including deep fried foods, chips,
  pizza and pies
- oils such as coconut and palm
- snack foods such as potato chips, chocolate,
  cookies and cakes

Make every effort to reduce your intake of saturated fats by eating less of the foods listed previously, and substituting with unsaturated fats whenever possible. For example:

Instead of:	Substitute:
Butter	monounsaturated spread (canola margarine)
Shortening/lard	polyunsaturated or monounsaturated oil
Regular milk	1% or skim milk
Fatty meat	smaller amounts of leaner cuts, such as London broil, flank steak and center loin pork chops
Regular ice cream	one of the many low fat varieties on the market
Regular cheese	low fat and reduced fat alternatives

WHAT FAT IS THAT?

The fat in our food is composed of different types of fatty acids. Depending on which fatty acids predominate, we identify the fat as either saturated, monounsaturated or polyunsaturated. Instead of using the saturated foods listed in the left-hand column below, try one of the monounsaturated or polyunsaturated alternatives listed in the middle and right-hand columns.

Instead of (Saturated)	Use this . . . (Monounsaturated)	Or this: (Polyunsaturated)
Butter	Canola margarine	Polyunsaturated margarines

Instead of (Saturated)	Use this . . . (Monounsaturated)	Or this: (Polyunsaturated)
	Olive margarine	(such as light tub margarines)
Shortening	Canola oil or margarine	Sunflower oil
	Olive oil or margarine	Safflower oil
	Canola margarine	Soybean oil
	Olive margarine	Light tub margarines
Palm oil	Peanut oil	Soybean oil
Coconut oil	Avocado oil	Walnut oil
	Peanut oil	Hazelnut oil
Cocoa butter	Canola margarine	Light tub margarines
	Olive margarine	

6. USE LESS SALT

Much of the salt we eat isn't from what we add ourselves: It's from salt already existing in foods. Bread and butter or margarine, for example, contributes much of the salt we eat. Low salt breads are rather untasty, but low salt butter and margarines are easy to find on supermarket shelves and aren't noticeably different in taste.

High-sodium foods include:

- canned, bottled and packet soups
- sauces, meal and gravy bases, bouillon
- ham, bacon, sausages and other delicatessen meats
- pizza, pot pies, fried chicken and other convenience foods
- pickles, chutneys, olives
- snack foods such as potato chips, pretzels, nachos, popcorn and salted nuts

7. CONSUME ALCOHOL IN MODERATION

There is no doubt that we all should avoid large quantities of alcohol, but several studies suggest that a moderate alcohol intake can offer a protective effect against heart disease.

People who drink one or two servings of alcohol per day, but not necessarily every day, show a reduced risk of heart disease, and the effect is greatest among those people with other risk factors for heart disease. Alcohol's effect may be because it increases the level of "good" HDL cholesterol. Antioxidant substances in red wine that reduce the oxidation of "bad" LDL cholesterol are also thought to be involved.

Please note: Three or more drinks per day actually increases the risk of death!

WHAT'S A SERVING OF ALCOHOL?

Here's how to measure one portion of alcohol:
- beer: 12 ounces
- wine: 5 ounces
- liquor: 1½ ounces

---

8. INCLUDE NUTS IN YOUR DIET

Nuts are a food that many people enjoy but few people eat regularly—a situation that needs to change! Large studies in recent years have found a strong link between higher consumption of nuts and reduced risk of heart disease. Nuts contain a very favorable mix of fatty acids that have a positive effect on blood fat levels.

Nuts are also a good source of other nutrients thought to protect against heart disease including vitamin E, folate (also called folic acid), copper and magnesium.

Because they are so nutrient and energy dense, you only need to eat nuts in small quantities. So sitting down to a bowl of nuts may not be such a good idea if you are trying to lose weight, but consuming small amounts of nuts regularly is quite healthy. Try:

- chopped almonds or pecans in granola
- a snack of nuts and dried fruit
- toasted cashews to top off a stir-fry
- a handful of pine nuts or sunflower seeds scattered over a salad

9. USE LOW FAT DAIRY PRODUCTS

Dairy foods are a great source of calcium, which our bodies need for strong bones and teeth. Luckily, calcium-rich, low fat flavored milks, puddings, yogurt, ice cream and mousse make great-tasting snacks and desserts!

Men and premenopausal women should aim to consume 1000 mg (milligrams) of calcium each day. After menopause, an optimal intake for women is 1200 mg a day. To get these amounts you'd need to eat at least three to four 1-cup servings of a low fat milk product daily.

One percent and nonfat milk supplies as much (and usually more) calcium as whole milk so is entirely suitable for those people who want to increase their calcium intake.

- 1 cup of 1% milk contains 300 mg of calcium and only 2½ grams of fat.
- 1 cup of whole milk contains 291 mg of calcium and 8 grams of fat.

■

EXPERTS RECOMMEND WHOLE MILK FOR CHILDREN UNDER AGE 2.

■

10. ALLOW YOURSELF A TREAT

We're meant to enjoy our food! So allow yourself to indulge in a little of whatever strikes your fancy—just ask yourself first whether it's what you really want.

- your favorite cheese and crackers
- a hot dog at the football game
- bacon and eggs on Sundays
- pizza on Friday night
- a slice of cake at a celebration
- chocolate chip cookies with a friend

■

THE MESSAGE FOR HEART DISEASE PREVENTION:
EAT A LOW FAT (AND LOW SATURATED FAT),
HIGH CARBOHYDRATE, HIGH FIBER AND LOW G.I. DIET
MOST OF THE TIME!

■

Chapter 11

CHECK THE LABEL FOR FAT

NUTRITION INFORMATION

WHICH FOODS ARE MOST FATTENING?

COUNTING THE CALORIES IN OUR NUTRIENTS

*U*se the numbers on the nutrition information panel to check the fat content of products when you're shopping.

NUTRITION INFORMATION

	per serving	per 100 grams
Energy	121 calories	486 calories
Protein	2.8 g	11.3 g
Fat	6.0 g	24.0 g
Carbohydrate total	14.1 g	56.3 g
Sugars	0.5 g	2.0 g

Across a range of products aim to buy those with less than 10 grams fat per 100 grams of food. In the example above, the fat content is 24 grams per 100 grams, or 24 percent fat. When the fat content is high, as this is, check the ingredient list for the type of fat:

Ingredients: wheat flour, vegetable oil (palm), tomato powder, salt, skim milk powder, yeast.

The main source of fat in this product is vegetable oil, which is specified as palm oil. From the table on page 48 we can see that palm oil is high in saturated fatty acids, so it would be best to choose another product with less saturated fat.

ARE YOU REALLY CHOOSING LOW FAT?

There's a trick to food labels that is worth being aware of when shopping for low fat foods. These food labeling specifications guidelines were enacted by the United States Department of Agriculture (USDA) in 1994:

Free: Contains a tiny or insignificant amount of fat, cholesterol, sodium, sugar or calories; less than 0.5 grams (g) of fat per serving.

Low fat: Contains no more than 3 g of fat per serving.

Reduced/Less/Fewer: These diet products must contain 25% less of a nutrient than the regular product.

Light/Lite: These diet products contain ⅓ fewer calories than, or ½ the fat of, the original product.

Lean: Meats with "lean" on the label contain less than 10 g of fat, 4 g of saturated fat, and 95 milligrams (mg) of cholesterol per serving.

Extra lean: These meats have less than 5 g of fat, 2 g of saturated fat and 95 mg of cholesterol per serving.

WHICH FOODS ARE MOST FATTENING?

Let's compare two everyday foods that are almost "pure" in a nutritional sense.

3 teaspoons of sugar	versus	1 teaspoon of butter
(almost pure carbohydrate)		(almost pure fat)

They contain virtually the same number of calories.

46 calories	versus	45 calories

This means that you can eat three times the volume of sugar as you could butter for the same number of calories! Look at these other examples:

- A small grilled T-bone steak (about the size of a slice of bread) has the same calories as 3 medium potatoes.
- 3 slices of bread, thickly buttered, are equivalent to 6 slices of bread with no butter.
- 4 Oreos have more calories than a carton of 2% chocolate milk.
- Eating 1 piece of breaded, fried chicken at lunch is the caloric equivalent of 6 slices of bread (without butter).
- For every 1 cup of fried rice you eat you could eat 2 cups of boiled rice.
- And if you're feeling extra hungry next time you stop for a coffee, consider that 1 glazed doughnut has the calories of 3 slices of lightly buttered cinnamon-raisin toast!

In every case the highest fat foods have the highest calorie counts. Because carbohydrate has about half the calories of fat, it is safer to eat more carbohydrate-rich food. What's more, your body is more likely to store fat and burn carbohydrate so the calories contribute more to your "spread" when they come from fat.

COUNTING THE CALORIES IN OUR NUTRIENTS

All foods contain calories. Often the caloric content of a food is considered a measure of how fattening it is. Of all the nutrients in food that we consume, carbohydrate yields the fewest calories per gram.

carbohydrate	4 calories per gram
protein	4 calories per gram
alcohol	7 calories per gram
fat	9 calories per gram

Chapter 12

7 DAYS OF HEART-HEALTHY EATING

*T*his week of menus shows you how to achieve a healthy heart diet with a low G.I. You can use the menus for ideas for your own meal choices or follow them closely to try out the low G.I. diet. Each menu is:

- **low in fat, especially saturated fat.** We've kept the total amount of fat down to provide less than 30 per cent of total calories, according to current recommendations. Saturated fat content is less than 20 grams per day.
- **low in calories.** These menus provide a total daily calorie intake of between 1400 and 1700 calories, which is a minimum amount for most

people. Be guided by your appetite to adjust quantities to suit yourself.

- high in carbohydrate with a low glycemic index. The carbohydrate content of these menus provides at least 50 percent of total calorie intake. This means at least 200 g of carbohydrate each day. The emphasis is on low G.I. carbohydrate choices.

Generally, beverages are included only where they make a significant nutrient or calorie contribution. Supplement the menus with a range of fluids such as water, tea, coffee, herbal tea, mineral water, soda with lemon or lime juice.

We list the recipe ideas for dishes marked with an asterisk on pages 65 to 67.

MONDAY

G.I.:	48
TOTAL ENERGY:	1500 cal.
SATURATED FAT:	7 g
CARBOHYDRATE:	239 g
FIBER:	40 g

Breakfast:
One cup All Bran with extra fiber, 1 small banana, 8 ounces 1% milk. Add 1 slice pumpernickel bread toast with 1 tablespoon light margarine (tub margarine) and a cup of tea or coffee.

Lunch:
A sandwich made from 2 slices of 100% stone-ground whole wheat bread, 3 ounces tuna and 1 tablespoon mayonnaise. Finish off with 4 ounces unsweetened canned peaches, and water or decaffeinated diet beverage.

Snack:
One oatmeal cookie and lemon tea

Dinner:
Two cups minestrone soup (homemade or canned), 2 ounces toasted pita, large mixed salad with fat free dressing. Water.

Night snack:
Four ounces low fat yogurt and ¾ cup fresh fruit salad

TUESDAY

G.I:	45
TOTAL ENERGY:	1500 cal.
SATURATED FAT:	12 g
CARBOHYDRATE:	228 g
FIBER:	19 g

Breakfast:
Two slices of 100% stoneground whole wheat toast with 4 tablespoons light ricotta cheese. Finish off with 1 small pear and 1 cup of hot chocolate made with 1% milk.

Lunch:
Try a sandwich made with 2 slices pumpernickel bread, 1 ounce of boiled ham and 1 ounce reduced-fat Cheddar cheese and 2 crispy pickle spears on the side. Finish with ¾ cup fresh fruit salad and water or decaffeinated diet beverage.

Afternoon snack:
One small low fat apple-cinnamon muffin

Dinner:
Four ounces Barbecued beef kebabs with ¾ cup Quick Rice Combo*. Finish with large tossed salad with fat-free dressing and beverage.

Night snack:
One-half cup low fat ice cream

*See recipe on page 66.

WEDNESDAY

G.I.:	43
TOTAL ENERGY:	1450 cal.
SATURATED FAT:	10 g
CARBOHYDRATE:	218 g
FIBER:	29 g

Breakfast:
One cup old-fashioned oatmeal made with 8 ounces 1% milk. Add ½ grapefruit, tea or coffee.

Lunch:
Two slices 100% stoneground whole wheat bread spread with 2 tablespoons natural peanut butter and 1 tablespoon all-fruit jelly. Finish with 1 cup grapes and water or decaffeinated diet beverage.

Afternoon snack:
Eight ounces fat-free fruited yogurt

Dinner:
Vegetarian Chili Fajita* with large tossed salad with fat-free dressing and water.

Night snack:
One ounce dry-roasted almonds and 1 cup of tea

*See recipe on page 66.

THURSDAY

G.I.:	46
TOTAL ENERGY:	1600 cal.
SATURATED FAT:	9 g
CARBOHYDRATE:	207g
FIBER:	42 g

Breakfast:
Toast 2 slices 100% stoneground whole wheat bread and top with 1 tablespoon of light (tub) margarine. Add 1 soft boiled egg, 1 medium peach, and cup of tea or coffee.

Lunch:
Two cups lentil soup (commercial or homemade) with tossed salad made with 2 tablespoons vinaigrette. Finish off with water or tea.

Afternoon snack:
An orange

Dinner:
One salmon cake* served with 1 cup frozen vegetable medley, 1 cup rice pilaf, and beverage.

Night snack:
One-half cup fat-free chocolate pudding

*See recipe on page 66.

FRIDAY

G.I.:	41
TOTAL ENERGY:	1400 cal.
SATURATED FAT:	11 g
CARBOHYDRATE:	226 g
FIBER:	15 g

Breakfast:
   One cup Special K with 8 ounces 1% milk and ½ banana. Tea or coffee.

Lunch:
   Sandwich made with 2 slices sourdough rye bread, 2 ounces smoked salmon and 1 tablespoon light cream cheese. Add 1 cup tomato, cucumber and onion salad with 2 tablespoons reduced-fat Italian dressing and water to drink.

Afternoon snack:
   One oatmeal cookie and 6 ounces nonfat fruited yogurt.

Dinner:
   One-and-one-half cups Easy Creamy Pasta* with tomato sauce, ½ cup green beans and 1 small baked apple with cinnamon for dessert. Top off with water or decaffeinated diet beverage.

Night snack:
   One-half cup low fat frozen yogurt (soft serve)

*See recipe on page 65.

SATURDAY

G.I.:	45
TOTAL ENERGY:	1650 cal.
SATURATED FAT:	15 g
CARBOHYDRATE:	236 g
FIBER:	27g

Breakfast:
Three 4-inch buckwheat pancakes, 1 tablespoon strawberry jam, 2 strips bacon and one small apple. Coffee or tea.

Lunch:
Inside a 2-ounce tortilla wrap 1 cup raw spinach, ½ cup diced tomato, 2 ounces turkey, 1 ounce cheese and 2 tablespoons light mayonnaise. Finish off with a large pear and water.

Afternoon snack:
One medium apple

Dinner:
Four ounces London broil, 1 medium sweet potato, 1 cup steamed broccoli with 1 teaspoon light (tub) margarine and a beverage.

Night snack:
Eight ounces apple juice with 3 Social Tea biscuits

SUNDAY

G.I.:	46
TOTAL ENERGY:	1600 cal.
SATURATED FAT:	13 g
CARBOHYDRATE:	181 g
FIBER:	21 g

Breakfast:
Three-quarters cup fresh fruit salad, 4 ounces low
fat fruited yogurt, 2 ounces apple cinnamon muffin. Tea or coffee.

Lunch:
Two slices pumpernickel bread, a 2-egg omelet
with diced tomatoes and shallots, and 2 tablespoons shredded Cheddar cheese. Add a tossed
green salad with fat free dressing and beverage.

Afternoon snack:
One banana

Dinner:
Broil a 6-ounce fish fillet (such as sole, flounder,
orange roughy or catfish) drizzled with one tablespoon olive oil, lemon juice, salt and pepper. Serve
with 6 ounces canned new potatoes and 1 cup (12
spears) asparagus or other seasonal vegetables.
Top off with cup of lemon tea.

Night snack:
Two ounces trail mix.

Chapter 13

QUICK MEAL IDEAS

EASY CREAMY PASTA

VEGETARIAN CHILI FAJITA

SALMON CAKES

QUICK RICE COMBO

BARBECUED BEEF KEBABS

*T*hese recipe ideas are used in the previous menu plans. The quantities are only a rough guide and can easily be adjusted to taste.

EASY CREAMY PASTA

Cook 8 ounces broad fettucine noodles according to box instructions. Combine ¼ cup of part-skim ricotta, ¼ cup of nonfat plain yogurt, ¼ cup of grated parmesan and 1 tablespoon of margarine. Stir this mixture through the drained pasta, adding some sautéed onion and garlic for extra flavor if desired. A quick topping idea: commercial pasta sauce.

SERVES 4.

VEGETARIAN CHILI FAJITA

Sauté a diced onion, a clove of crushed garlic, and thin strips of green pepper. Add 4 thinly sliced mushrooms and oregano to taste and cook 5 minutes. Stir in a small can of red kidney beans. Sprinkle a 2-ounce tortilla with ½ cup of shredded reduced fat cheddar or Monterey jack cheese. Spoon the bean mixture onto the tortilla and fold it over to enclose the ingredients. Pour about ½ cup of salsa or picante sauce over tortilla and top with another ½ cup of cheese. Bake 10–15 minutes in hot oven.

SERVES 4.

■

SALMON CAKES

Combine a 6-ounce can of salmon with ½ onion (finely diced), ½ cup mashed potato, 2 teaspoons chopped parsley and 1 egg. Shape into patties and fry in a pan sprayed with cooking spray.

SERVES 2.

■

QUICK RICE COMBO

Fry 2 strips of trimmed diced bacon, 1 diced small red pepper, 2 chopped shallots and 1 cup of frozen peas. Add 2 cups of cooked Uncle Ben's Converted rice, drizzle with soy sauce and serve.

SERVES 4.

BARBECUED BEEF KEBABS

Marinate approximately 1 pound of cubed beef (e.g. top round or sirloin) in ½ cup red wine, 1 tablespoon vinegar, 1 tablespoon olive oil, 1 teaspoon Worcestershire sauce, 2 tablespoons ketchup, crushed garlic and black pepper. Thread the meat cubes onto the skewer alternately with mushrooms and pepper and onion strips. Grill or barbecue and serve with Quick Rice Combo.

SERVES 4.

■

Chapter 14

A G.I. SUCCESS STORY

$\mathcal{T}$o help illustrate how a low G.I. diet can improve your heart disease risk factors, dietitian Johanna Burani, M.S., R.D., C.D.E., offers this real-life example from her own practice. Many of Johanna's patients have lost weight, controlled their diabetes and gained overall better health by choosing a low G.I. way of life.

CASE STUDY:
"JAY"

Age: 66
Height: 5'10"
Weight: 171 pounds (healthy weight range for his height)

BACKGROUND:

Jay is a retired letter carrier who used to smoke and drink until he quit some 15 years ago. He hates to exercise. Jay suffers from Type 2 diabetes and has elevated blood fats. He has already undergone successful triple bypass surgery.

Jay's typical diet before surgery:
Breakfast: Fried eggs, Taylor ham, home fries, and several cups of coffee (with half and half and sugar) and buttered toast
Lunch: A salami sandwich on a hard roll, donut and Coke
Snack: Several pieces of coffee cake with coffee
Dinner: Steak, baked potato with butter, salad, apple pie a la mode, Coke
Late night snack: Three or four scoops of ice cream (large bowl)

JAY'S "BEFORE" NUTRITIONAL ANALYSIS:

Calories: 4250
Carbohydrate: 447 g (42%)
Protein: 265 g (25%)
Fat: 156 g (33%)
G.I.: 72

Johanna's nutritional assessment:
To maximize the health benefits of his successful heart surgery, it was paramount for Jay to decrease his total caloric intake, take a serious look at his

dietary sources of fat (specifically saturated fat) and
find ways to incorporate a minimum of five servings
of fruits and vegetables into his diet every day.

G.I.-specific counseling:

Jay's carbohydrate intake (nearly 1800 calories) came
almost exclusively from refined starches (such as
white bread, rolls, baked goods and sugar). The rapid
digestion of these foods kept Jay hungry, so he ate
large meals and snacks. He didn't think there was
any problem with this way of eating since he wasn't
overweight. The more calories he consumed, however, the greater his cholesterol and saturated fat intake
was, which eventually clogged three of his arteries,
necessitating bypass surgery.

  Solution: The low G.I., high-fiber foods that he
would incorporate into his diet would enable Jay to
feel full longer—as the higher-fat foods did previously—but without the negative impact on his once-
compromised heart's health. A low G.I. diet would
have the added benefit of improving Jay's diabetes
control.

Jay's new, low G.I. menu:

Johanna put Jay on a 2,800-calorie-a-day, low G.I.
meal plan for a 4-week transitional period, after
which Jay followed a 2,000-calorie-a-day menu eating meals such as these:

Breakfast: Two slices sourdough rye toast with 1
   tablespoon light (tub) margarine, Egg Beater
   omelet with mushrooms and onions, small glass of
   grapefruit juice, reduced caffeine coffee with Equal
   and fat-free half and half

Snack: Eight-ounce glass 1% milk, (with 2 ounces
   cold coffee), 2 or 3 graham crackers

Lunch: A double-decker sandwich: (3 slices sourdough rye bread, 2 slices boiled ham, 2 slices reduced-fat cheese, large sliced cucumber), fatfree, no-sugar-added cooked butterscotch pudding, seltzer

Snack: Decaffeinated Diet Coke

Dinner: One cup rice pilaf, 6 ounces broiled scallops in wine and lemon sauce, 1 cup cooked wax beans, a handful of grapes, seltzer

Snack: Low fat apple-cinnamon muffin, herbal tea

JAY'S "AFTER" NUTRITIONAL ANALYSIS:

Calories: 2000
Carbohydrate: 287 g (56%)
Protein: 110 g (24%)
Fat: 50 g (24%)
G.I.: 52

Jay's winning results:

It's been more than two years since Jay's bypass surgery. He continues to follow the low fat, high fiber, low G.I. guidelines that Johanna gave him after his surgery. He's also maintained a healthy weight, which is currently 172½ pounds. His blood pressure remains good without medication and his blood sugars have been excellent long enough for his doctor to suggest that he try cutting back from two pills a day to just one. He successfully completed his cardiac rehabilitation program and only needs to visit his cardiologist once a year.

Jay's comments:
"I feel great; nothing bothers me. I hate to exercise, but my wife hollers at me if I don't, so I take a short walk every day."

Chapter 15

YOUR QUESTIONS
ANSWERED

HEART DISEASE, WEIGHT LOSS AND
LOW G.I. DIETS

CAN YOU EAT ALL THE CARBOHYDRATES
YOU WANT?

IS SUGAR FATTENING?

AND MORE . . .

*I have heart disease and my doctor has told me to
lose weight. How can a high carbohydrate–low G.I.
diet help me shed pounds?*

Because low G.I. diets lower insulin levels, over
the long term you'll burn more—and store less—fat.
(Insulin determines how much fat we store and
burn.) And . . .

- You're less likely to overeat low G.I. carbohydrates, because they're bulky and filling.
  Consider them natural appetite suppressants!
- A low G.I. diet offers you plenty of food choices, so you're less likely to feel deprived. Unlike
  diets that restrict certain foods, a low G.I. diet is
  easy to live with.

Can I still lose weight eating as much carbohydrate as I want?

Possibly not. We recommend a high carbohydrate intake and a low fat intake. While carbohydrate is not usually stored as fat, if you are eating more total energy than your body requires, then the carbohydrate will be used as a source of fuel in preference to fat. This would have the effect of limiting the breakdown of body fat stores. The idea is to eat enough energy in total to satisfy your appetite (using low G.I. foods helps) and nutritional requirements, but not more than you need. An increase in your activity level will help burn up body fat as it is used as an additional fuel.

I've always heard that sugar is fattening. Is it?

No. Sugar has no special fattening properties—in fact, it is no more likely to be turned into fat than any other carbohydrate. Sugar, which you'll often find in foods high in calories and fat may sometimes seem to be "turned into fat," but it's the total number of calories you're consuming rather than the sugar in those calorie dense foods that may contribute to new stores of fat.

Why are diets that disregard widely accepted nutritional guidelines so fashionable right now?

Several best-selling books have been published promoting high protein diets and generating a lot of publicity. They have been seized upon as a viable weight loss panacea. But the fact is: Diets that limit major food groups do not work over the long haul.

What are the side effects of a high protein diet?

The body cannot process large quantities of protein, so excess waste is produced that can overburden the kidneys. Not only can some high protein diets make existing kidney problems worse, but they also can cause mild renal failure to progress faster. Some high protein diets are also harmful for elderly people and anyone with high blood pressure or diabetes. High protein, high fat diets can lead to high cholesterol, heart disease, and increase the risk of heart attack. Further, some high protein diets reduce the intake of important vitamins, minerals, fiber and trace elements. They also lack fiber, which may lead to constipation.

Overweight people with heart disease need to shed pounds. Why do people on high protein diets lose weight?

Because they make people lose water weight. Overweight people need to lose body fat—not muscle or water. And the way to do this is by eating a balanced diet of low G.I. carbohydrates and burning more calories than we take in.

Chapter 16

YOUR HEART-HEALTHY, LOW G.I. PANTRY

BREADS

BREAKFAST CEREALS

RICE AND GRAINS

LEGUMES

VEGETABLES

FRUITS

DAIRY FOODS

MEATS

FISH

SEAFOOD

USEFUL FLAVORINGS, SAUCES AND DRESSINGS

WHAT TO KEEP IN THE REFRIGERATOR AND FREEZER

*N*othing affects our day-to-day food choices as much as what we have in the cupboard. Use these ideas as the basis of your shopping list.

BREADS

We recommend eating all types of bread, but the best choices are the whole grain varieties. If you're the only one in the family who enjoys whole grain breads, keep a loaf in the freezer and pull out slices as you need them.

- 100% stoneground whole wheat
- Rye
- Banana bread
- Chapati (baisen)
- Natural Ovens 100% Whole Grain**
- Natural Ovens Happiness**
- Natural Ovens Hunger Filler**
- Natural Ovens Natural Wheat**
- Sourdough
- Sourdough rye
- Whole grain pumpernickel
- Whole wheat pita

**Natural Ovens breads are available in the United States through mail order. See "For More Information" on page 106 for ordering information.

BREAKFAST CEREALS

Cereals enriched with psyllium, when eaten as part of a low fat diet, lower levels of "bad" cholesterol, but maintain "good" cholesterol levels.

- Kellogg's All-Bran with extra fiber
- Kellogg's Bran Buds with Psyllium
- Muesli (low fat varieties, read the labels)
- Rolled or old-fashioned oats
- Oat bran
- Rice bran
- Oatmeal

■ ■ ■

RICE AND GRAINS

- Pearled barley
- Basmati rice, brown or long-grain rice
- Uncle Ben's Converted Rice
- Pasta, fresh or dried, of various shapes and flavors
- Noodles

LEGUMES

- Cooked lentils (red or brown), chickpeas, split peas
- Dried lentils, chickpeas, cannellini beans
- A variety of canned legumes (kidney beans, mixed beans, baked beans, lentils, chickpeas, black beans, pinto beans, butter beans, broad beans, chana dal)

VEGETABLES

All vegetables are good for you—fresh, frozen and canned. Raw salad vegetables are available partially prepared to make a quick addition to the meal. Here are some low G.I. veggie varieties:

- Peas
- Sweet corn
- Sweet potato
- Canned new potatoes
- Carrots

Other canned vegetables such as tomatoes, asparagus, peas, corn, beets, mushrooms and canned mixed veggies are handy to boost the vegetable content of a meal. Other convenient products are:

- Tomato paste
- Tomato puree
- Tomato pasta sauces (in jars)
- Frozen vegetables

FRUITS

The lowest G.I. fresh fruit choices include:

- Cherries
- Grapefruit
- Pears
- Apples
- Plums
- Peaches
- Oranges
- Grapes
- Kiwi
- Dried fruits, such as dried apricots, fruit medley, raisins, prunes etc.
- Canned fruit cocktail, peaches, pears (in fruit juice), or natural applesauce
- Unsweetened fruit juices are also suitable as long as you don't drink them to excess, so drink no more than 1 or 2 cups a day.

DAIRY FOODS

- Shelf-stable skim milk or skim milk powder— easy to use in cooking
- Canned evaporated skim milk

- Cook 'n' Serve Sugar Free Pudding and Pie Filling

USEFUL FLAVORINGS, SAUCES AND DRESSINGS

- Spices—curry powder, cumin, turmeric, mustard, and so on
- Herbs—oregano, basil, thyme, etc.
- Bottled minced ginger, chili and garlic
- Sauces (such as soy, chili, oyster, hoi sin, teriyaki, Worcestershire)
- Bouillon
- Low oil salad dressings

WHAT TO KEEP IN THE REFRIGERATOR AND FREEZER

Meats
- Any meat trimmed of all visible fat
- Low fat ground meat
- Skinless chicken or turkey
- Canadian bacon
- Lean cold meats—ham, corned beef, pastrami, turkey, chicken breast or roast beef

Seafood and shellfish
We recommend all types of fresh fish. Some of the best choices for prepared items include:

- Canned fish such as salmon, mackerel, tuna, herring and sardines
- Smoked fish, including cod and salmon

- Frozen fish products that contain a minimal amount of saturated fat (check the labels carefully!)

It's fine to eat most seafood and shellfish regularly; just steer clear of battered or crumbed varieties or foods in creamy sauces. Calamari is okay, but don't eat it more than once a week if you have high cholesterol.

Dairy foods
- Skim or 1% milk
- Nonfat plain yogurt
- Light fruited yogurt
- Low fat ice cream
- Frozen low fat yogurt, sorbet, gelato
- Low fat block and processed cheese (check the label for those which are less than 10 percent fat.)
- Margarine labeled "polyunsaturated" or "monounsaturated" (and prefeably salt reduced).

Cheese
- Low fat processed slices
- Reduced fat Swiss (such as Jarlsberg Light)
- Grated parmesan
- 1% or 2% cottage or part-skim ricotta cheese

Vegetables and legumes
- Frozen peas, corn, spinach, carrots, and others

Fruit
- Frozen berries and melon balls

Chapter 17

CUTTING THE FAT: YOUR A TO Z GUIDE

*A*s we have said constantly throughout this book, it is important to eat a high carbohydrate and low fat diet. The following practical tips that we have set out in an easy A to Z format will help you reduce the fat content of some of your favorite recipes while lowering their glycemic index.

Alcohol Although excessive alcohol consumption can be fattening, as an ingredient in a recipe, alcohol itself won't create a high calorie dish. Alcohol evaporates during cooking, so you lose the calories and are left with the flavor. A little wine in a sauce can give a delicious flavor, and sherry in an Asian style marinade is essential.

Bacon Bacon is a valuable ingredient in many dishes because of the flavor it offers. You can make a little bacon go a long way by trimming off all fat and chopping it finely. Lean ham is often a more economical and leaner way to go. In casseroles and soups, a ham or bacon bone imparts a fine flavor without much fat.

Cheese At around 30 percent fat (23 percent of it saturated), cheese can contribute quite a lot of fat to a recipe. Although there are a number of fat-reduced cheeses available, many of these lose a lot in flavor for a small reduction in fat. It is worth comparing fat per ounce between brands to find the tastiest one with the lowest fat content. Alternatively, a sprinkle of a grated, very tasty cheese or Parmesan may do the job.

Part skim ricotta and cottage cheeses are lower fat alternatives to butter on a sandwich. It's worth trying some fresh part skim ricotta from a deli—you may find the texture and flavor more acceptable than that of the ricotta available in containers in the supermarket. Flavored cottage cheeses are ideal low fat toppings for crackers. Try ricotta in lasagna instead of a creamy white sauce.

Cream and sour cream Keep to very small amounts as these are high in saturated fat. Substitute nonfat sour cream, which tastes very similar to the full fat variety. A 16 ounce container of heavy cream can be poured into ice-cube trays and frozen providing small servings of cream easily when you need it. Adding one ice-cube block (1 oz.) of cream to a dish adds only 5½ grams of fat.

Dried beans, peas and lentils These are all low in fat and very nutritious. Incorporating them in a recipe, perhaps as partial substitution of meat, will lower the fat content of the finished product. Canned beans, chickpeas and lentils are now widely available. They are very convenient to use and a great time saver. They are comparable in food value to the dried ones that you soak and cook yourself.

Eggs Be conscious of eggs in a recipe as they can add fat. Sometimes just the beaten egg white can be substituted for the whole egg, or use real egg substitute.

Filo pastry Unlike most other pastry, filo (also known as phyllo) is low in fat. To keep it that way, brush between the sheets with skim milk instead of melted butter when you prepare it. Look for it in the freezer section of the supermarket with other prepared pastry and use it as a pie filling or a strudel wrap.

Grilling Grill or broil tender cuts of meat, chicken and fish rather than fry. Marinating first will add flavor, moisture and tenderness.

Health food stores Health food stores can be traps for the unwary. Check out the high fat ingredients, such as hydrogenated vegetable oil, nuts, coconut and palm kernel oil in the products such as granola bars, fruit bars and "healthy" cakes (even if made with whole wheat flour) that they stock on their shelves.

Ice cream A source of carbohydrate, calcium, riboflavin, retinol and protein and low fat varieties have lower G.I. values—definitely a nutritious and icy treat.

Jam A tablespoon of jam on toast contains far fewer calories than a pat of butter. So, enjoy your jam and give fat the flick!

Keep jars of minced garlic, chili or ginger in the refrigerator to spice up your cooking in an instant.

Lemon juice Try a fresh squeeze with ground black pepper on vegetables rather than a pat of butter. Lemon juice provides acidity that slows gastric emptying and lowers the glycemic index.

Milk Many people dislike skim milk, particularly when they taste it on its own or in their coffee! However, you can use skim milk in a recipe and no one will notice—and the fat savings is great. For convenience you might want to keep powdered skim milk in the pantry, which can be made up to the desired quantity when you need it. It will taste more like fresh milk if you mix the powder and water according to directions and refrigerate the milk overnight before using it. Ultra-pasteurized (or shelf stable) milk is handy in the cupboard, too.

Nuts They are valuable for their content of vitamin E, but they are also high in fat. To keep the fat content of a recipe low, the quantity of nuts has to be small.

Oil Most of our recipes call for no more than 2 teaspoons of oil. Any polyunsaturated or monounsaturated oil is suitable. Cooking spray or brushing oil lightly over the base of the pan is ideal. If you find the amount of oil insufficient, cover your pan, or add a few drops of water and use steam to cook the ingredients without burning. It is a good idea to invest in a nonstick frying pan if you don't have one!

Pasta A food to eat more of and a great source of carbohydrate and B vitamins. Fresh or dried, the preparation is easy. Just boil in water until just tender or "al dente," drain and top with a dollop of pesto, a tomato sauce or a sprinkle of Parmesan and pepper. There are many wonderful pasta cookbooks now available, and it's definitely worth investing in one to find all sorts of exciting ways to prepare this fabulous low G.I. food. Pasta may appear in your menu as a side dish to meat, as noodles in soup, as a meal in itself with vegetables or sauce or even as an ingredient in a dessert.

Questions Ask your dietitian for more recipe ideas. (See page 105 for guidance on finding a dietitian near you.)

Reduce the fat content of ground beef by browning it in a nonstick pan, then placing the meat in a colander and pouring boiling water through it to wash away the fat. Return to the pan to continue cooking. It is a good idea to buy the better quality ground beef with less fat.

Stock If you are prepared to go to the effort of making your own stock—good for you! Prepare it in advance, refrigerate it then skim off the accumulated fat from the top. Prepared stock is available in long-life cartons and cans in the supermarket. Stock cubes are another alternative. Look for brands that have reduced salt.

To sauté Heat the pan first, brush with the recommended amount of oil (or less), add the food and cook, stirring lightly over a gentle heat.

Underlying the need for fat is a need for taste. Be creative with other flavorings.

Vinegar A vinaigrette dressing (1 tablespoon vinegar and 2 teaspoons of oil) with your salad can lower the blood sugar response to the whole meal by up to 30 percent. The best types of vinegars for this purpose are red or white wine vinegar, or use lemon juice.

Weighing What's the weight of the meat you're buying? Start noticing the weight that appears on the butcher's scales or package label and consider how many servings it will give you. With a food such as steak, that is basically all edible meat, 4 to 5 ounces per serving is sufficient. One pound is more than enough for four portions. Choose lean cuts of meat and trim away the fat before cooking or before you put it away. Alternate meat or chicken with fish once or twice a week.

Yogurt Yogurt is a valuable food in many ways. It is a good source of calcium, "friendly bacteria," protein and riboflavin, and unlike milk, is suitable for those people who are lactose intolerant. Low fat plain yogurt is a suitable substitute for sour cream. If using yogurt in a hot sauce or casserole, add it at the last minute and do not let it boil, or it will curdle. It is best if you can bring the yogurt to room temperature before adding to the hot dish. To do this, mix a small amount of yogurt with a little sauce from the dish, then stir this mixture back into the bulk of the sauce.

Zero fat Eating zero fat is unhealthy, so speak with a dietitian about how to get just the right amount you need. Our bodies need essential fatty acids that can't be synthesized and must be supplied in the diet. Fat does add flavor—use it to your advantage.

Chapter 18

HOW TO USE
THE G.I. TABLE

---

*T*he following table is an A to Z listing of the glycemic index of commonly eaten foods in the United States and Canada. Approximately 300 different foods are listed, including some new values for foods tested only recently.

The G.I. value shown next to each food is the average for that food using glucose as the standard (i.e., glucose has a G.I. value of 100, with other foods rated accordingly). The average may represent the mean of 10 studies of that food worldwide or only 2 to 4 studies. In a few instances, American data are different from the rest of the world and we show that data rather than the average. Rice and oatmeal fall into this category.

To check on a food's glycemic index, simply look

for it by name in the alphabetic list. You may also find it under a food type—fruit, cookies.

Included in the tables is the carbohydrate (CHO) and fat content of a sample serving of the food. This is to help you keep track of the amount of fat and carbohydrate in your diet. The sample serving is not the recommended serving—it is just an example of a serving. The glycemic index does not depend on your serving size because it is a ranking of the glycemic effect of foods using carbohydrate-equivalent portion sizes. You can eat more of a low G.I. food or less of a high G.I. food and achieve the same blood sugar levels.

Remember when you are choosing foods, their G.I. is not the only aspect to consider. Throughout this guide we have stressed the need to minimize your saturated fat intake and eat a balanced variety of foods. If you can't find the G.I. value of a food you eat on many occasions, please write or e-mail us, and we'll give you an estimate of its G.I. value.

Address your letter to:

Associate Professor Jennie Brand-Miller
Human Nutrition Unit
Department of Biochemistry
University of Sydney, NSW, 2006
Fax 61(02) 9351 6022
E-mail j.brandmiller@biochem.usyd.edu.au

Chapter 19

THE GLYCEMIC INDEX TABLE

A–Z OF FOODS WITH GLYCEMIC INDEX, CARBOHYDRATE & FAT

Food	Glycemic Index	Fat (g per svg.)	CHO (g per svg.)
Agave nectar (90% fructose syrup), 1 tablespoon	11	0	16
All-Bran with extra fiber™, Kellogg's, breakfast cereal, ½ cup, 1 oz.	51 (av)	1	22
Angel food cake, ½ cake, 1 oz.	67	trace	17
Apple, 1 medium, 5 ozs.	38 (av)	0	18
Apple, dried, 1 oz.	29	0	24
Apple juice, unsweetened, 1 cup, 8 ozs.	40	0	29
Apple cinnamon muffin, from mix, 1 muffin	44	5	26
Apricots, fresh, 3 medium, 3 ozs.	57	0	12
canned, light syrup, 3 halves	64	0	14
dried, 5 halves	31	0	13
Apricot jam, no added sugar, 1 tablespoon	55	0	17
Apricot and honey muffin, low fat, from mix, 1 muffin	60	4	27
Bagel, 1 small, plain, 2.3 ozs.	72	1	38
Baked beans, ½ cup, 4 ozs.	48 (av)	1	24
Banana bread, 1 slice, 3 ozs.	47	7	46
Banana, raw, 1 medium, 5 ozs.	55 (av)	0	32
Banana, oat and honey muffin, low fat from mix, 1 muffin	65	4	27
Barley, pearled, boiled, ½ cup, 2.6 ozs.	25 (av)	0	22
Basmati white rice, boiled, 1 cup, 6 ozs.	58	0	50
Beets, canned, drained, ½ cup, 3 ozs.	64	0	5
Black bean soup, ½ cup, 4 ½ ozs.	64	2	19
Black beans, boiled, ¾ cup, 4.3 ozs.	30	1	31
Black bread, dark rye, 1 slice, 1.7 ozs.	76	1	18
Blackeyed peas, canned, ½ cup, 4 ozs.	42	1	16
Blueberry muffin, 1 muffin, 2 ozs.	59	4	27
Bran			
All-Bran with extra fiber™, Kellogg's, ½ cup, 1 oz.	51	1	20

Food	Glycemic Index	Fat (g per svg.)	CHO (g per svg.)
Bran Buds with Psyllium™, Kellogg's, ⅓ cup, 1 oz.	45	1	24
Bran Flakes, Post, ⅔ cup, 1 oz.	74	1	22
Multi-Bran Chex™, General Mills, 1 cup, 2.1 ozs.	58	1.5	49
Oat bran, 1 tablespoon	55	1	7
Oat bran muffin, 2 ozs.	60	4	28
Rice bran, 1 tablespoon	19	2	5
Breads			
Dark rye, Black bread, 1 slice, 1.7 ozs.	76	1	18
Dark rye, Schinkenbrot, 1 slice, 2 ozs.	86	1	22
French baguette, 1 oz.	95	1	15
Gluten-free bread, 1 slice	90	1	18
Hamburger bun, 1 prepacked bun, 1½ ozs.	61	2	22
Kaiser roll, 1, 2 ozs.	73	2	34
Light deli (American) rye, 1 slice, 1 oz.	68	1	16
Melba toast, 6 pieces, 1 oz.	70	2	23
Natural Ovens 100% Whole Grain, 1 slice, 1.2 ozs.	51	0	17
Natural Ovens Hunger Filler, 1 slice, 1.2 ozs.	59	0	16
Natural Ovens Natural Wheat, 1 slice, 1.2 ozs.	59	0	16
Natural Ovens Happiness, 1 slice, 1.1 oz.	63	0	15
Pita bread, whole wheat, 6½ inch loaf, 2 ozs.	57	2	35
Pumpernickel, whole grain, 1 slice, 1 oz.	51	1	15
Rye bread, 1 slice, 1 oz.	65	1	15
Sourdough, 1 slice, 1½ ozs.	52	1	20
Sourdough rye, Arnold's, 1 slice, 1½ ozs.	57	1	21
White, 1 slice, 1 oz.	70 (av)	1	12
100% stoneground whole wheat, 1 slice, 1½ ozs.	53	1	15
Whole wheat, 1 slice, 1 oz.	69 (av)	1	13
Bread stuffing from mix, 2 ozs.	74	5	13
Breakfast cereals			
All-Bran with extra fiber™, Kellogg's, ½ cup, 1 oz.	51	1	20
Bran Buds with Psyllium™, Kellogg's, ½ cup, 1 oz.	45	1	24
Bran Flakes, Post, ⅔ cup, 1 oz.	74	1	22
Cheerios™, General Mills, 1 cup, 1 oz.	74	2	23
Cocoa Krispies™, Kellogg's, 1 cup, 1 oz.	77	1	27
Corn Bran™, Quaker Crunchy, ¾ cup, 1 oz.	75	1	23
Corn Chex™, Nabisco, 1 cup, 1 oz.	83	0	26
Corn Flakes™, Kellogg's, 1 cup, 1 oz.	84 (av)	0	24
Cream of Wheat, instant, 1 packet, 1 oz.	74	0	21

Food	Glycemic Index	Fat (g per svg.)	CHO (g per svg.)
Cream of Wheat, old fashioned, ¾ cup, cooked, 6 ozs.	66	0	21
Crispix™, Kellogg's, 1 cup, 1 oz.	87	0	25
Frosted Flakes™, Kellogg's, ¾ cup, 1 oz.	55	0	28
Golden Grahams™, General Mills, ¾ cup, 1.6 ozs.	71	1	25
Grapenuts™, Post, ¼ cup, 1 oz.	67	1	27
Grapenuts Flakes™, Post, ¾ cup, 1 oz.	80	1	24
Life™, Quaker, ¾ cup, 1 oz.	66	1	25
Muesli, natural muesli, ⅔ cup, 1½ ozs.	56	3	28
Muesli, breakfast cereal, toasted, ⅔ cup, 2 ozs.	43	10	41
Multi-Bran Chex™, General Mills, 1 cup, 2.1 ozs.	58	1.5	49
Oat bran, raw, 1 tablespoon	55	1	7
Oat bran™, Quaker Oats, ¾ cup, 1 oz.	50	1	23
Oatmeal (made with water), old fashioned, cooked, ½ cup, 4 ozs.	49 (av)	1	12
Oats, 1-minute, Quaker Oats, 1 cup, cooked	66	2	25
Puffed Wheat™, Quaker, 2 cups, 1 oz.	67	0	22
Raisin Bran™, Kellogg's, ¾ cup, 1 oz.	73	0	32
Rice bran, 1 tablespoon	19	2	5
Rice Chex™, General Mills, 1¼ cups, 1 oz.	89	0	27
Rice Krispies™, Kellogg's, 1¼ cups, 1 oz.	82	0	26
Shredded wheat, spoonsize, ⅔ cup, 1.2 ozs.	58	0	27
Shredded Wheat™, Post, breakfast cereal, 1 oz.	83	1	23
Smacks™, Kellogg's, ¾ cup, 1 oz.	56	1	24
Special K™, Kellogg's, 1 cup, 1 oz.	66	0	22
Team Flakes™, Nabisco, ¾ cup, 1 oz.	82	0	25
Total™, General Mills, ¾ cup, 1 oz.	76	1	24
Weetabix™, 2 biscuits, 1.2 ozs.	75	1	28
Buckwheat groats, cooked, ½ cup, 2.7 ozs.	54 (av)	1	20
Bulgur, cooked, ⅔ cup, 4 ozs.	48 (av)	0	23
Bun, hamburger, 1 prepacked bun, 1.7 ozs.	61	2	22
Butter beans, boiled, ½ cup, 4 ozs.	31 (av)	0	16
Cakes			
Angel food cake, 1 slice, 1⁄12 cake, 1 oz.	67	trace	17
Banana bread, 1 slice, 3 ozs.	47	7	46
Pound cake, homemade, 1 slice, 3 ozs.	54	15	42
Sponge cake, 1 slice, 1⁄12 cake, 2 ozs.	46	4	32
Capellini pasta, cooked, 1 cup, 6 ozs.	45	1	53
Cantaloupe, raw, ¼ small, 6½ ozs.	65	0	16

Food	Glycemic Index	Fat (g per svg.)	CHO (g per svg.)
Carrots, peeled, boiled, canned, ½ cup, 2.4 ozs.	49	0	3
Carrots, peeled, boiled, canned, ½ cup, 2.4 ozs.	49	0	3
Cereal grains			
Barley, pearled, boiled, ½ cup, 2.6 ozs.	25 (av)	0	22
Bulgur, cooked, ½ cup, 3 ozs.	48 (av)	0	17
Couscous, cooked, ½ cup, 3 ozs.	65 (av)	0	21
Corn			
Cornmeal, whole grain, from mix, cooked, ⅓ cup, 1.4 ozs.	68	1	30
Sweet corn, canned, drained, ½ cup, 3 ozs.	55 (av)	1	15
Taco shells, 2 shells, 1 oz.	68	5	17
Rice			
Basmati, white, boiled, 1 cup, 6 ozs.	58	0	50
Brown, 1 cup, 6 ozs.	55 (av)	0	37
Converted™, Uncle Ben's, 1 cup, 6 ozs.	44	0	38
Instant, cooked, 1 cup, 6 ozs.	87	0	37
Long grain, white, 1 cup, 6 ozs.	56 (av)	0	42
Parboiled, 1 cup, 6 ozs.	48	0	38
Rice cakes, plain, 3 cakes, 1 oz.	82	1	23
Short grain, white, 1 cup, 6 ozs.	72	0	42
Chana dal, ½ cup, 4 ozs.	8	3	28
Cheerios™, General Mills, breakfast cereal, 1 cup, 1 oz.	74	2	23
Cherries, 10 large cherries, 3 ozs.	22	0	10
Chickpeas (garbanzo beans),canned, drained, ½ cup, 4 ozs.	42	2	15
boiled, ½ cup, 3 ozs.	33 (av)	2	23
Chocolate butterscotch muffin, low fat from mix, 1 muffin	53	4	29
Chocolate, bar, 1½ ozs.	49	14	26
Chocolate Flavor, Nestle Quik™ (made with water), 3 teaspoons	53	0	14
Coca-Cola™, soft drink, 1 can	63	0	39
Cocoa Krispies™, Kellogg's, breakfast cereal, 1 cup, 1 oz.	77	1	27
Corn			
Cornmeal, cooked from mix, ⅓ cup, 1.4 ozs.	68	1	30
Sweet corn, canned and drained, ½ cup, 3 ozs.	55 (av)	1	15
Corn Bran™, Quaker Crunchy, breakfast cereal, ¾ cup, 1 oz.	75	1	23
Corn Chex™, General Mills, breakfast cereal, 1 cup, 1 oz.	83	0	26
Corn chips, 1 oz.	72	10	16
Corn Flakes™, Kellogg's, breakfast cereal, 1 cup, 1 oz.	84 (av)	0	24
Cornmeal, from mix, cooked, ⅓ cup, 1.4 ozs.	68	1	30

Food	Glycemic Index	Fat (g per svg.)	CHO (g per svg.)
Cookies			
Graham crackers, 4 squares, 1 oz.	74	3	22
Milk Arrowroot, 3 cookies, ½ oz.	69	2	9
Oatmeal, 1 cookie, ⅔ oz.	55	3	12
Shortbread, 4 small cookies, 1 oz.	64	7	19
Social Tea™ biscuits, Nabisco, 4 cookies, ⅔ oz.	55	3	13
Vanilla wafers, 7 cookies, 1 oz.	77	4	21
see also Crackers			
Couscous, cooked, ⅔ cup, 4 ozs.	65 (av)	0	21
Crackers			
Crispbread, 3 crackers, ⅔ oz.	81	0	15
Kavli™ All Natural Whole Grain Crispbread, 4 wafers, 1 oz.	71	1	16
Premium soda crackers, saltine, 8 crackers, 1 oz.	74	3	17
Rice cakes, plain, 3 cakes, 1 oz.	82	1	23
Ryvita™ Tasty Dark Rye Whole Grain Crisp Bread, 2 slices, ⅔ oz.	69	1	16
Stoned wheat thins, 3 crackers, ½ oz.	67	2	15
Water cracker, Carr's, 3 king size crackers, ⅘ oz.	78	2	18
Cream of Wheat, instant, 1 packet, 1 oz.	74	0	21
Cream of Wheat, old fashioned, ¾ cup, cooked, 6 ozs.	66	0	21
Crispix™, Kellogg's, breakfast cereal, 1 cup, 1 oz.	87	0	25
Croissant, medium, 1.2 ozs.	67	14	27
Custard, ½ cup, 4.4 ozs.	43	4	24
Dairy foods and nondairy substitutes			
Ice cream, 10% fat, vanilla, ½ cup, 2.2 ozs.	61 (av)	7	16
Ice milk, vanilla, ½ cup, 2.2 ozs.	50	3	15
Milk, whole, 1 cup, 8 ozs.	27 (av)	9	11
skim, 1 cup, 8 ozs.	32	0	12
chocolate flavored, 1%, 1 cup, 8 ozs.	34	3	26
Pudding, ½ cup, 4.4 ozs.	43	4	24
Soy milk, 1 cup, 8 ozs.	31	7	14
Tofu frozen dessert (nondairy), low fat, ½ cup, 2 ozs.	115	1	21
Yogurt			
nonfat, fruit flavored, with sugar, 8 ozs.	33	0	30
nonfat, plain, artificial sweetener, 8 ozs.	14	0	17
nonfat, fruit flavored, artificial sweetener, 8 ozs.	14	0	16
Dates, dried, 5, 1.4 ozs.	103	0	27
Doughnut with cinnamon and sugar, 1.6 ozs.	76	11	29
Fanta™, soft drink, 1 can	68	0	47

Food	Glycemic Index	Fat (g per svg.)	CHO (g per svg.)
Fava beans, frozen, boiled, ½ cup, 3 ozs.	79	0	17
Fettucine, cooked, 1 cup, 6 ozs.	32	1	57
Fish sticks, frozen, oven-cooked, fingers, 3½ ozs.	38	14	24
Flan cake, ½ cup, 4 ozs.	65	5	23
French baguette bread, 1 oz.	95	0	15
French fries, large, 4.3 ozs.	75	22	46
Frosted Flakes™, Kellogg's, breakfast cereal, ¾ cup, 1 oz.	55	0	28
Fructose, pure, 3 packets	23 (av)	0	10
Fruit cocktail, canned in natural juice, ½ cup, 4 ozs.	55	0	15
Fruits and fruit products			
Agave nectar (90% fructose syrup), 1 tablespoon	11	0	16
Apple, 1 medium, 5 ozs.	38 (av)	0	18
Apple, dried, 1 oz.	29	0	24
Apple juice, unsweetened, 1 cup, 8 ozs.	40	0	29
Apricots, fresh, 3 medium, 3.3 ozs.	57	0	12
canned, light syrup, 3 halves	64	0	19
dried, 1 oz.	31	0	13
Apricot jam, no added sugar, 1 tablespoon	55	0	17
Banana, raw, 1 medium, 5 ozs.	55 (av)	0	32
Cantaloupe, raw, ¼ small, 6½ ozs.	65	0	16
Cherries, 10 large, 3 ozs.	22	0	10
Dates, dried, 5, 1.4 ozs.	103	0	27
Fruit cocktail, canned in natural juice, ½ cup, 4 ozs.	55	0	15
Grapefruit, raw, ½ medium, 3.3 ozs.	25	0	5
Grapefruit juice, unsweetened, 1 cup, 8 ozs.	48	0	22
Grapes, green, 1 cup, 3 ozs.	46 (av)	0	15
Kiwi, 1 medium, raw, peeled, 2½ ozs.	52 (av)	0	8
Mango, 1 small, 5 ozs.	55 (av)	0	19
Marmalade, 1 tablespoon	48	0	17
Orange, navel, 1 medium, 4 ozs.	44 (av)	0	10
Orange juice, 1 cup, 8 ozs.	46	0	26
Papaya, ½ medium, 5 ozs.	58 (av)	0	14
Peach, fresh, 1 medium, 3 ozs.	28	0	7
canned, natural juice, ½ cup, 4 ozs.	30	0	14
canned, light syrup, ½ cup, 4 ozs.	52	0	18
canned, heavy syrup, ½ cup, 4 ozs.	58	0	26
Pear, fresh, 1 medium, 5 ozs.	38 (av)	0	21
canned in pear juice, ½ cup, 4 ozs.	44	0	13

Food	Glycemic Index	Fat (g per svg.)	CHO (g per svg.)
Pineapple, fresh, 2 slices, 4 ozs.	66	0	10
Pineapple juice, unsweetened, canned, 8 ozs.	46	0	34
Plums, 1 medium, 2 ozs.	39 (av)	0	7
Raisins, ¼ cup, 1 oz.	64	0	28
Strawberry jam, 1 tablespoon	51	0	18
Watermelon, 1 cup, 5 ozs.	72	0	8
Gatorade™ sports drink, 1 cup, 8 ozs.	78	0	14
Glucose powder, 2½ tablets	102	0	10
Gluten-free bread, 1 slice, 1 oz.	90	1	18
Golden Grahams™, General Mills, ¾ cup, 1.6 ozs.	71	1	25
Granola Bars™, Quaker Chewy, 1 oz.	61	2	23
Gnocchi, cooked, 1 cup, 5 ozs.	68	3	71
Graham crackers, 4 squares, 1 oz.	74	3	22
Grapefruit, raw, ½ medium, 3.3 ozs.	25	0	5
Grapefruit juice unsweetened, 1 cup, 8 ozs.	48	0	22
Grapenuts™, Post, breakfast cereal, ¼ cup, 1 oz.	67	1	27
Grapenuts Flakes™, Post, breakfast cereal, ¾ cup, 1 oz.	80	1	24
Grapes, green, 1 cup, 3.3 ozs.	46 (av)	0	15
Green pea soup, canned, ready to serve, 1 cup, 9 ozs.	66	3	27
Hamburger bun, 1 prepacked bun, 1½ ozs.	61	2	22
Honey, 1 tablespoon	58	0	16
Ice cream, 10% fat, vanilla, ½ cup, 2.2 ozs.	61 (av)	7	16
Ice milk, vanilla, ½ cup, 2.2 ozs.	50	3	15
Isostar, 1 cup, 8 ozs.	73	0	18
Jelly beans, 10 large, 1 oz.	80	0	26
Kaiser rolls, 1 roll, 2 ozs.	73	2	34
Kavli™ All Natural Whole Grain Crispbread, 4 wafers, 1 oz.	71	1	16
Kidney beans, red, boiled, ½ cup, 3 ozs.	27 (av)	0	20
Kidney beans, red, canned and drained, ½ cup, 4.3 ozs.	52	0	19
Kiwi, 1 medium, raw, peeled, 2½ ozs.	52 (av)	0	8
Kudos Granola Bars™ (whole grain), 1 bar, 1 oz.	62	5	20
Lactose, pure, ⁷⁄₁₀ oz.	46 (av)	0	10
Lentil soup, Unico, canned, 1 cup, 8 ozs.	44	1	24
Lentils, green and brown, boiled, ½ cup, 3 ozs.	30 (av)	0	16
Lentils, red, boiled, 1.4 cup, 4 ozs.	26 (av)	0	27
Life™, Quaker, breakfast cereal, ¾ cup, 1 oz.	66	1	25
Life Savers™, roll candy, 6 pieces, peppermint	70	0	10
Light deli (American) rye bread, 1 slice, 1 oz.	68	1	16

Food	Glycemic Index	Fat (g per svg.)	CHO (g per svg.)
Lima beans, baby, frozen, ½ cup, 3 ozs.	32	0	17
Linguine pasta, thick, cooked, 1 cup, 6 ozs.	46 (av)	1	56
Linguine pasta, thin, cooked, 1 cup, 6 ozs.	55 (av)	1	56
M&M's Chocolate Candies Peanut™, 1.7 oz. package	33	13	30
Macaroni and Cheese Dinner™, Kraft packaged, cooked, 1 cup, 7 ozs.	64	17	48
Macaroni, cooked, 1 cup, 6 ozs.	45	1	52
Maltose (maltodextrin), pure, 2½ teaspoons	105	0	10
Mango, 1 small, 5 ozs.	55 (av)	0	19
Marmalade, 1 tablespoon	48	0	17
Mars Almond Bar™, 1.8 ozs.	65	12	31
Melba toast, 6 pieces, 1 oz.	70	2	23
Milk, whole, 1 cup, 8 ozs.	27 (av)	9	11
skim, 1 cup, 8 ozs.	32	0	12
chocolate flavored, 1%, 1 cup, 8 ozs.	34	3	26
Milk Arrowroot, 3 cookies, ½ oz.	63	2	9
Millet, cooked, ½ cup, 4 ozs.	71	1	2
Muesli, breakfast cereal, toasted, ⅔ cup, 2 ozs.	43	10	41
Muesli, non-toasted, ⅔ cup, 1½ ozs.	56	3	28
Multi-Bran Chex™, General Mills, 1 cup, 2.1 ozs.	58	1.5	49
Muffins			
Apple cinnamon, from mix, 1 muffin, 2 ozs.	44	8	33
Apricot and honey, low fat, from mix, 1 muffin	60	4	27
Banana, oat and honey, low fat, from mix, 1 muffin	65	4	27
Blueberry, 1 muffin, 2 ozs.	59	4	27
Chocolate butterscotch, low fat, from mix, 1 muffin	53	4	29
Oat and raisin, low fat, from mix, 1 muffin	54	3	28
Oat bran, 1 muffin, 2 ozs.	60	4	28
Mung beans, boiled, ½ cup, 3½ ozs.	38	1	18
Natural Ovens 100% Whole Grain bread, 1 slice, 1.2 ozs.	51	0	17
Natural Ovens Hunger Filler bread, 1 slice, 1.2 ozs.	59	0	16
Natural Ovens Natural Wheat bread, 1 slice, 1.2 ozs.	59	0	16
Natural Ovens Happiness bread, 1 slice, 1.1 ozs.	63	0	15
Navy beans, boiled, ½ cup, 3 ozs.	38 (av)	0	
Nutella™ (spread), 2 tablespoons, 1 oz.	33	9	19
Oat and raisin muffin, low fat from mix, 1 muffin	54	3	28
Oat bran, 1 tablespoon	55	1	7

Food	Glycemic Index	Fat (g per svg.)	CHO (g per svg.)
Oat bran™, Quaker Oats, breakfast cereal, ¾ cup, 1 oz.	50	1	23
Oat bran, 1 muffin, 2 ozs.	60	4	28
Oatmeal (made with water), old fashioned, cooked, 1 cup, 8 ozs.	49	2	26
Oatmeal cookie, 1, ⅗ oz.	55	3	12
Oats, 1-minute, Quaker Oats, 1 cup, cooked	66	2	25
Orange, navel, 1 medium, 4 ozs.	44 (av)	0	10
Orange syrup, diluted, 1 cup	66	0	20
Orange juice, 1 cup, 8 ozs.	46	0	26
Papaya, ½ medium, 5 ozs.	58 (av)	0	14
Parsnips, boiled, ½ cup, 2½ ozs.	97	0	15
Pasta			
Capellini, cooked, 1 cup, 6 ozs.	45	1	53
Fettucine, cooked, 1 cup, 6 ozs.	32	1	57
Gnocchi, cooked, 1 cup, 5 ozs.	68	3	71
Linguine thick, cooked, 1 cup, 6 ozs.	46 (av)	1	56
Linguine thin, cooked, 1 cup, 6 ozs.	55 (av)	1	56
Macaroni, cooked, 1 cup, 5 ozs.	45	1	52
Macaroni & Cheese Dinner™, Kraft, packaged, cooked, 1 cup, 7 ozs.	64	17	48
Ravioli, meat-filled, cooked, 1 cup, 9 ozs.	39	8	32
Spaghetti, white, cooked, 1 cup, 6 ozs.	41 (av)	1	52
Spaghetti, whole wheat, cooked, 1 cup, 6 ozs.	37 (av)	1	48
Spirali, durum, cooked, 1 cup, 6 ozs.	43	1	56
Star Pastina, cooked, 1 cup, 6 ozs.	38	1	56
Tortellini, cheese, cooked, 8 ozs.	50	6	26
Vermicelli, cooked, 1 cup, 6 ozs.	35	0	42
Pastry, flaky, ⅛ of double crust, 2 ozs.	59	15	24
Pea soup, split with ham, canned, 1 cup, Wil-Pak Foods, 5½ ozs.	66	7	56
Peach, fresh, 1 medium, 3 ozs.	28	0	7
canned, heavy syrup, ½ cup, 4 ozs.	58	0	26
canned, light syrup, ½ cup, 4 ozs.	52	0	18
canned, natural juice, ½ cup, 4 ozs.	30	0	14
Peanuts, roasted, salted, ½ cup, 2½ ozs.	14 (av)	38	16
Pear, fresh, 1 medium, 5 ozs.	38 (av)	0	21
canned in pear juice, ½ cup, 4 ozs.	44	0	13
Peas, green, fresh, frozen, boiled, ½ cup, 2.7 ozs.	48 (av)	0	11
Peas dried, boiled, ½ cup, 2 ozs.	22	0	7

Food	Glycemic Index	Fat (g per svg.)	CHO (g per svg.)
Pineapple, fresh, 2 slices, 4 ozs.	66	0	10
Pineapple juice, unsweetened, canned, 8 ozs.	46	0	34
Pinto beans, canned, ½ cup, 4 ozs.	45	1	18
Pinto beans, soaked, boiled, ½ cup, 3 ozs.	39	0	22
Pita bread, whole wheat, 6½ inch loaf, 2 ozs.	57	2	35
Pizza, cheese and tomato, 2 slices, 8 ozs.	60	22	56
Plums, 1 medium, 2 ozs.	39 (av)	0	7
Popcorn, light, microwave, 2 cups (popped)	55	3	12
Potatoes			
Desirée, peeled, boiled, 1 medium, 4 ozs.	101	0	13
French fries, large, 4.3 ozs.	75	26	49
instant mashed potatoes, Carnation Foods™, ½ cup, 3½ ozs.	86	2	14
new, unpeeled, boiled, 5 small (cocktail), 6 ozs.	62 (av)	0	23
new, canned, drained, 5 small, 6 ozs.	61	0	23
red-skinned, peeled, boiled, 1 medium, 4 ozs.	88 (av)	0	15
red-skinned, baked in oven (no fat), 1 medium, 4 ozs.	93 (av)	0	15
red-skinned, mashed, ½ cup, 4 ozs.	91 (av)	0	16
red-skinned, microwaved, 1 medium, 4 ozs.	79	0	15
sweet potato, peeled, boiled, ½ cup mashed, 3 ozs.	54 (av)	0	20
white-skinned, peeled, boiled, 1 medium, 4 ozs.	63 (cv)	0	24
white-skinned, with skin, baked in oven (no fat), 1 medium, 4 ozs.	85 (av)	0	30
white-skinned, mashed, ½ cup, 4 ozs.	70 (av)	0	20
white-skinned, with skin, microwaved, 1 medium, 4 ozs.	82	0	29
Sebago, peeled, boiled, 1 medium, 4 ozs.	87	0	13
Potato chips, plain, 14 pieces, 1 oz.	54 (av)	11	15
Pound cake, 1 slice, homemade, 3 ozs.	54	15	42
Power Bar™, Performance, Chocolate, 1 bar	58	2	45
Premium saltine crackers, 8 crackers, 1 oz.	74	3	17
Pretzels, 1 oz.	83	1	22
Puffed Wheat™, Quaker, breakfast cereal, 2 cups, 1 oz.	67	0	22
Pumpernickel bread, whole grain, 2 slices	51	2	30
Pumpkin, peeled, boiled, mashed, ½ cup, 4 ozs.	75	0	6
Raisins, ¼ cup, 1 oz.	64	0	28
Raisin Bran™, Kellogg's, breakfast cereal, ¾ cup, 1.3 ozs.	73	0	32
Ravioli, meat-filled, cooked, 1 cup, 9 ozs.	39	8	32
Rice			
Basmati, white, boiled, 1 cup, 7 ozs.	58	0	50

Food	Glycemic Index	Fat (g per svg.)	CHO (g per svg.)
Brown, 1 cup, 6 ozs.	55 (av)	0	37
Converted™, Uncle Ben's, 1 cup, 6 ozs.	44	0	38
Instant, cooked, 1 cup, 6 ozs.	87	0	37
Long grain, white, 1 cup, 6 ozs.	56 (av)	0	42
Parboiled, 1 cup, 6 ozs.	48	0	38
Rice bran, 1 tablespoon	19	2	5
Rice cakes, plain, 3 cakes, 1 oz.	82	1	23
Short grain, white, 1 cup, 6 ozs.	72	0	42
Rice Chex™, General Mills, breakfast cereal, 1¼ cups, 1 oz.	89	0	27
Rice Krispies™, Kellogg's, breakfast cereal, 1¼ cups, 1 oz.	82	0	26
Rice vermicelli, cooked, 6 ozs.	58	0	48
Roll (bread), Kaiser, 1 roll, 2 ozs.	73	2	39
Romano (cranberry) beans, boiled, ½ cup, 3 ozs.	46	0	21
Rutabaga, peeled, boiled, ½ cup, 2.6 ozs.	72	0	3
Rye bread, 1 slice, 1 oz.	65	1	15
Ryvita™ Tasty Dark Rye Whole Grain Crisp Bread, 2 slices, ⅔ oz.	69	1	16
Sausages, smoked link, pork and beef, fried, 2½ ozs.	28	29	5
Semolina, cooked, ⅔ cup, 6 ozs.	55	0	17
Shortbread, 4 small cookies, 1 oz.	64	7	19
Shredded Wheat™, Post, breakfast cereal, 1 oz.	83	1	23
Shredded wheat, 1 biscuit, ⅚ oz.	62	0	19
Skittles Original Fruit Bite Size Candies™, 2.3 oz. pk.	70	3	59
Smacks™, Kellogg's, breakfast cereal, ¾ cup, 1 oz.	56	1	24
Snickers™, 2.2 oz. bar	41	15	36
Social Tea™ biscuits, Nabisco, 4 cookies, ⅔ oz.	55	3	13
Soft drink, Fanta™, 1 can, 12 ozs.	68	0	47
Soups			
Black bean soup, ½ cup, 4½ ozs.	64	2	19
Green pea soup, canned, ready to serve, 1 cup, 9 ozs.	66	3	27
Lentil soup, Unico, canned, 1 cup, 8 ozs.	44	1	24
Pea soup, split, with ham, Wil-Pak Foods, 1 cup, 5½ ozs.	66	7	56
Tomato soup, canned, 1 cup, 9 ozs.	38	4	33
Sourdough bread, 1 slice, 1½ ozs.	52	1	20
Rye bread, Arnold's, 1 slice, 1½ ozs.	57	1	21
Soy beans, boiled, ½ cup, 3 ozs.	18 (av)	7	10
Soy milk, 1 cup, 8 ozs.	31	7	14
Spaghetti, white, cooked, 1 cup	41 (av)	1	52
Spaghetti, whole wheat, cooked, 1 cup, 5 ozs.	37 (av)	1	48

Food	Glycemic Index	Fat (g per svg.)	CHO (g per svg.)
Special K™, Kellogg's, breakfast cereal, 1 cup, 1 oz.	66	0	22
Spirali, durum, cooked, 1 cup, 6 ozs.	43	1	56
Split pea soup, 8 ozs.	60	4	38
Split peas, yellow, boiled, ½ cup, 3½ ozs.	32	0	21
Sponge cake plain, 1 slice, 3 ½ ozs.	46	4	32
Sports drinks			
Gatorade™ 1 cup, 8 ozs.	78	0	14
Isostar, 1 cup, 8 ozs.	73	0	18
Sportsplus, 1 cup, 8 ozs.	74	0	17
Sports bars			
Power Bar™, Performance Chocolate Bar, 1 bar	58	2	45
Stoned wheat thins, 3 crackers, ⅔ oz.	67	2	15
Strawberry Nestle Quik™ (made with water), 3 teaspoons	64	0	14
Strawberry jam, 1 tablespoon	51	0	18
Sucrose, 1 teaspoon	65 (av)	0	4
Syrup, fruit flavored, diluted, 1 cup	66	0	20
Sweet corn, canned, drained, ½ cup, 3 ozs.	55 (av)	1	16
Sweet potato, peeled, boiled, ½ cup mashed, 3 ozs.	54 (av)	0	20
Taco shells, 2 shells, 1 oz.	68	5	17
Tapioca pudding, boiled with whole milk, 1 cup, 10 ozs.	81	13	51
Taro, peeled, boiled, ½ cup, 2 ozs.	54	0	23
Team Flakes™, Nabisco, breakfast cereal, ¾ cup, 1 oz.	82	0	25
Tofu frozen dessert, nondairy, low fat, 2 ozs.	115	1	21
Tomato soup, canned, 1 cup, 9 ozs.	38	4	33
Tortellini, cheese, cooked, 8 ozs.	50	6	26
Total™, General Mills, breakfast cereal, ¾ cup, 1 oz.	76	1	24
Twix Chocolate Caramel Cookie™, 2, 2 ozs.	44	14	37
Vanilla wafers, 7 cookies, 1 oz.	77	4	21
Vermicelli, cooked, 1 cup, 6 ozs.	35	0	42
Vitasoy™ Soy milk, creamy original, 1 cup, 8 ozs.	31	7	14
Waffles, plain, frozen, 4 inch square, 1 oz.	76	3	13
Water crackers, 3 king size crackers, ⅔ oz.	78	2	18
Watermelon, 1 cup, 5 ozs.	72	0	8
Weetabix™ breakfast cereal, 2 biscuits, 1.2 ozs.	75	1	28
White bread, 1 slice, 1 oz.	70 (av)	1	12
Whole wheat bread, 1 slice, 1 oz.	69 (av)	1	13
Yam, boiled, 3 ozs.	51	0	31

Food	Glycemic Index	Fat (g per svg.)	CHO (g per svg.)
Yogurt			
nonfat, fruit flavored, with sugar, 8 ozs.	33	0	30
nonfat, plain, artificial sweetener, 8 ozs.	14	0	17
nonfat, fruit flavored, artificial sweetener, 8 ozs.	14	0	16

GLYCEMIC INDEX TESTING

If you are a food manufacturer, you may be interested in having the glycemic index of some of your products tested on a fee-for-service basis. For more information, contact either:

> Glycaemic Index Testing Inc.
> 135 Mavety Street
> Toronto, Ontario
> Canada M6P 2L8
> E-mail: thomas.wolever@utoronto.ca

or

> Sydney University Glycaemic Index Research Service (SUGIRS)
> Department of Biochemistry
> University of Sydney
> NSW 2006 Australia
> Fax: (61) (2) 9351-6022
> E-mail: j.brandmiller@staff.usyd.edu.au

FOR MORE INFORMATION

REGISTERED DIETITIANS

Registered Dietitians (R.D.s) are nutrition experts who provide nutritional assessment and guidance and support for people with heart disease. Check for the initials "R.D." after the name to identify qualified dietitians who provide the highest standard of care to their clients. Glycemic index is part of their training so all dietitians should be able to help in applying the principles in this guide, but some dietitians do specialize in certain areas. If you want more detailed advice on glycemic index just ask the dietitian whether this is a specialty when you make your appointment.

Dietitians work in hospitals and often run their own private practices, as well. For a list of dietitians in your area, contact the American Dietetic Association (ADA) Consumer Nutrition Hotline (1-800-366-1655) or visit ADA's home page at the address below. You can also check the Yellow Pages under "Dietitians."

The American Dietetic Association
216 West Jackson Boulevard
Chicago, IL 60606
Phone: 1-800-877-1600
Fax: 1-312-899-1979
Web site: http://www.eatright.org/

PRIMARY CARE PHYSICIANS

If you have heart disease or think you may have it, keep in close contact with your primary care physician or heart specialist.

WEIGHT LOSS ORGANIZATIONS

To help you lose weight, check the Yellow Pages under "Weight Control Services." Be aware, however, that not all weight loss organizations are reputable. Check with your physician to make sure the group you'd like to join can help you lose weight safely.

HEART HELP

For more information about the prevention and treatment of stroke, heart disease and related conditions, contact:

The American Heart Association
7272 Greenville Avenue
Dallas, TX 75231
Phone: 1-800-AHA-USA1
Web site: http://www.americanheart.org

NATURAL OVENS ORDERING INFORMATION

Natural Ovens of Manitowoc
4300 County Trunk CR
P.O. Box 730
Manitowoc WI 54221-0730

Telephone: 1-800-772-0730
Fax: 920-758-2594
http://www.naturalovens.com/

ACKNOWLEDGMENTS

We would like to acknowledge the extraordinary efforts of Johanna Burani and Linda Rao, who adapted this book—and the other books in *The Glucose Revolution Pocket Guide* series—for North American readers. Together they have worked to ensure that every piece of information is accurate and appropriate for readers in the U.S. and Canada.

For more information about *The Glucose Revolution* and *The Glucose Revolution Pocket Guides*, visit **www.glucoserevolution.com**

ABOUT THE AUTHORS

Kaye Foster-Powell, B.Sc., M. Nutr. & Diet., is an accredited dietitian-nutritionist in both public and private practice in New South Wales, Australia. A graduate of the University of Sydney (B.Sc., 1987; Master of Nutrition and Dietetics, 1994), she has extensive experience in diabetes management and has researched practical applications of the glycemic index over the last five years. A co-author of *The Glucose Revolution* and all the titles in *The Glucose Revolution Pocket Guide* Series, she lives in Sydney, Australia.

Jennie Brand-Miller, Ph.D., Associate Professor of Human Nutrition in the Human Nutrition Unit, Department of Biochemistry, University of Sydney, Australia, is widely recognized as one of the world's leading authorities on the glycemic index. She received her B.Sc. (1975) and Ph.D. (1979) degrees from the Department of Food Science and Technology at the University of New South Wales, Australia. She is the editor of the *Proceedings of the Nutrition Society of Australia* and a member of the Scientific Consultative Committee of the Australian Nutrition Foundation. She has written more than 200 research papers, including 60 on the glycemic index of foods. A co-author of *The Glucose Revolution* and all the titles in *The Glucose Revolution Pocket Guide* Series, she lives in Sydney, Australia.

Anthony Leeds, M.D., is Senior Lecturer in the Department of Nutrition & Dietetics at King's College London. He graduated in medicine from the Middlesex Hospital Medical School, London, in 1971. He conducts research on carbohydrate and dietary fiber in relation to heart disease, obesity and diabetes, continues part-time medical practice and is a member of the European Association of Scientific Editors. He chairs the research ethics committee of King's College London and in 1999 was elected a Fellow of the Institute of Biology. He is a co-author of the U.K. edition of *The Glucose Revolution*.

Thomas M.S. Wolever, M.D., Ph.D., another of the world's leading researchers of the glycemic index, is Professor in the Department of Nutritional Sciences, University of Toronto, and a member of the Division of Endocrinology and Metabolism, St. Michael's Hospital, Toronto. He is a graduate of Oxford University (B.A., M.A., M.B., B.Ch., M.Sc., and D.M.) in the United Kingdom. He received his Ph.D. at the University of Toronto. His research since 1980 has focused on the glycemic index of foods and the prevention of type 2 diabetes. A co-author of *The Glucose Revolution* and all the titles in *The Glucose Revolution Pocket Guide* Series, he lives in Toronto, Canada.

Johanna Burani, M.S., R.D., C.D.E., is a registered dietitian and certified diabetes educator with more than 10 years experience in nutritional counseling. She specializes in designing individual meal plans based on low glycemic-index food choices. The adapter of *The Glucose Revolution* and co-adapter, with Linda Rao, of all the titles in *The Glucose Revolution Pocket Guide* Series, she is the author of seven books and professional manuals, and lives in Mendham, New Jersey.

Linda Rao, M.Ed., a freelance writer and editor, has been writing and researching health topics for the past 11 years. Her work has appeared in several national publications, including *Prevention* and *USA Today*. She serves as a contributing editor for *Prevention* Magazine and is the co-adapter, with Johanna Burani, of all the titles in *The Glucose Revolution Pocket Guide* Series. She lives in Allentown, Pennsylvania.

The Glucose Revolution begins here . . .

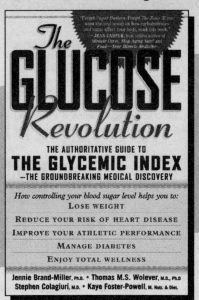

THE GLUCOSE REVOLUTION
THE AUTHORITATIVE GUIDE TO THE GLYCEMIC INDEX—
THE GROUNDBREAKING MEDICAL DISCOVERY

NATIONAL BESTSELLER!

"Forget *Sugar Busters*. Forget *The Zone*. If you want the real scoop on how carbohydrates and sugar affect your body, read this book by the world's leading researchers on the subject. It's the authoritative, last word on choosing foods to control your blood sugar."

—JEAN CARPER, best-selling author of *Miracle Brain, Miracle Cures, Stop Aging Now!* and *Food—Your Miracle Medicine*

ISBN 1-56924-660-2 • $14.95

. . . and continues with these other
Glucose Revolution Pocket Guides

The Glucose Revolution Pocket Guide to
LOSING WEIGHT

Eat yourself slim with low glycemic index foods

Not all foods are created equal when it comes to losing weight. The latest medical research shows that carbohydrates with a low glycemic index have special advantages because they fill you up and keep you satisfied longer. This pocket guide will help you eat yourself slim with low glycemic index foods and show you how low glycemic index foods make sustained weight loss possible. This guide also includes a 7-day low glycemic index plan for losing weight, G.I. success stories, and the glycemic index and fat and carbohydrate content of more than 300 foods and drinks.

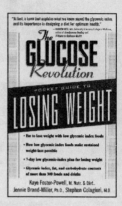

ISBN 1-56924-677-7 • $4.95

The Glucose Revolution Pocket Guide to
SPORTS NUTRITION

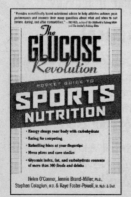

Eat to compete better than ever before.

Serious athletes and weekend warriors can gain a winning edge by manipulating the glycemic index of their diets. Now this at-a-glance guide shows how to use the glycemic index to boost athletic performance, enhance stamina, and prevent fatigue. Subjects covered include energy charging with carbohydrates, eating for competing, refueling hints, menu plans and case studies, and the glycemic index, fat and carbohydrate content of more than 300 foods and drinks.

ISBN 1-56924-676-9 • $4.95

The Glucose Revolution Pocket Guide to
DIABETES

Help control your diabetes with low glycemic index foods

Based on the most up-to-date information about carbohydrates, this basic guide to the glycemic index and diabetes allows people with type 1 and type 2 diabetes to make more informed choices about their diets. Topics covered include why many traditionally "taboo" foods don't cause the unfavorable effects on blood sugar levels they were believed to have, and why diets based on low G.I. foods improve blood sugar control. Also covered are how to include more of the right kinds of carbohydrates in your diet, the

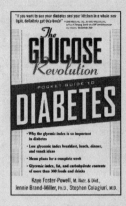

optimum diet for people with diabetes, practical hints for meal preparation and tips to help make the glycemic index work throughout the day, a week of low G.I. menus, G.I. success stories, and more.
ISBN 1-56924-675-0 • $4.95

The Glucose Revolution Pocket Guide to
SUGAR AND ENERGY

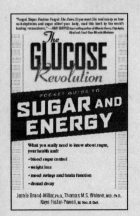

Sugar's off the black list—find out why

Based on the most up-to-date information about carbohydrates, this basic guide to the glycemic index dispels many common myths about sugar and why it's high time to get rid of the guilt. With evidence showing that restricting refined sugar in your diet may do more harm than good, the authors show you how to intelligently give in to your sugar cravings and regulate your sugar intake to control your blood sugar level and lose weight, with the glycemic index for nearly 150 foods.
ISBN 1-56924-641-6 • $4.95

The Glucose Revolution Pocket Guide to
THE TOP 100 LOW GLYCEMIC FOODS

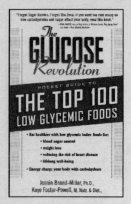

ISBN 1-56924-678-5 • $4.95

The best of the best in low glycemic index foods

The slow digestion and gradual rise and fall in blood sugar levels after a food with a low glycemic index has benefits for many people. Today we know the glycemic index of hundreds of different generic and name-brand foods, which have been tested following a standardized method. Now *The Top 100 Low Glycemic Foods* makes it easy to enjoy those slowly digested carbohydrates every day for better blood sugar control, weight loss, a healthy heart, and peak athletic performance.